Praise for
DOCTORED

A *New York Post* Best Book of 2014

"Bold and fascinating . . . [Jauhar] interweaves his personal story as well as anecdotes about his patients into a meticulously researched and painfully honest account of a profession."
—Suzanne Koven, *The Boston Globe*

"Arresting . . . Dr. Jauhar's book is often moving, especially when he focuses on his patients . . . This thoughtful telling provides a service in itself. Because the first step toward healing, of course, is getting a good diagnosis." —Susannah Meadows, *The New York Times*

"In this absorbing memoir-cum-analysis, Sandeep Jauhar traces his years as a fledgling cardiologist against the backdrop of a health-care system in peril . . . An impassioned call to action." —Barbara Kiser, *Nature*

"A compelling call for reform." —New York *Daily News*

"Sandeep Jauhar's *Doctored* is a passionate and necessary book that asks difficult questions about the future of medicine. The narrative is gripping, and the writing is marvelous. But it was the gravity of the problem—so movingly told—that grabbed and kept my attention throughout this remarkable work."
—Siddhartha Mukherjee, author of *The Emperor of All Maladies: A Biography of Cancer*

"Medicine's radical transformation in recent years has brought both incredible scientific advances and an increasingly dysfunctional health care system. *Doctored* takes us behind the façade and allows us to see the seamy underbelly. Jauhar's gift is to observe and to beautifully tell the stories. In doing so he leads us to a visceral understanding of what has gone wrong. *Doctored* is a manifesto for reform."

—Abraham Verghese, author of *Cutting for Stone*

"Sandeep Jauhar specializes in peeling back the veneer, revealing the discomfiting truths of today's medical world. He is unafraid to dig deeply and honestly, both within himself and within the medical profession. *Doctored* raises critical questions that twenty-first-century medicine must answer if it is to meet the needs of its patients as well as of its practitioners."

—Danielle Ofri, M.D., Ph.D., author of *What Doctors Feel: How Emotions Affect the Practice of Medicine*

"Sandeep Jauhar is a compelling storyteller, and *Doctored* gives us a fantastic tour through the seedy underworld of American medicine."

—Lisa Sanders, M.D., Assistant Professor, Yale School of Medicine, and author of *Every Patient Tells a Story*

"In this searing critique of overtreatment, cronyism and cover-your-ass medical care, a cardiologist confronts the 'collective malaise' infecting the American medical profession as he opens a vein to reveal his own complicity and shattered ideals. Jauhar offers, if not a cure, a prescription for restoring dignity to patient and healer alike."

—Nanette Varian, *More*

"*Doctored* hits home with its accounts of expensive, needless, even redundant tests and the staggering medical bills that they entail. With unsparing candor, the memoir describes [Jauhar's] own moral crisis as he reflects on the profession he so values. A major document in an ongoing discussion that no one with a heartbeat can ignore."

—*Barnes & Noble*

"A supremely well-written, thought-provoking memoir that strikes the perfect balance between ideas and sentiment."

—G. Sampath, *Mint* (India)

ALSO BY SANDEEP JAUHAR

Intern: A Doctor's Initiation

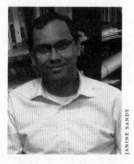

Sandeep Jauhar
DOCTORED

Sandeep Jauhar, M.D., Ph.D., is the director of the Heart Failure Program at Long Island Jewish Medical Center. He is the author of *Intern* and a contributing opinion writer for *The New York Times*. He lives on Long Island with his wife and their son and daughter.

DOCTORED

DOCTORED

The Disillusionment of an
American Physician

SANDEEP JAUHAR

Farrar, Straus and Giroux
New York

Farrar, Straus and Giroux
18 West 18th Street, New York 10011

Portions of this book originally appeared in different form in *The New York Times*, the *Los Angeles Times*, *The New England Journal of Medicine*, and the anthology *Becoming a Doctor* (W. W. Norton & Company, Inc., 2010).

The Library of Congress has cataloged the hardcover edition as follows:
Jauhar, Sandeep, 1968–
    Doctored : the disillusionment of an American physician / Sandeep
Jauhar. — First edition.
        p. ; cm.
    ISBN 978-0-374-14139-4 (hardback) — ISBN 978-1-4299-4584-4 (ebook)
    I. Title.
    [DNLM: 1. Jauhar, Sandeep, 1968– 2. Physicians—United States—
Autobiography. 3. Delivery of Health Care—trends—United States. WZ 100]

R153
610.92—dc23
[B]
                                                            2013041344

Paperback ISBN: 978-0-374-53533-9

Designed by Jonathan D. Lippincott

Farrar, Straus and Giroux books may be purchased for educational, business, or promotional use. For information on bulk purchases, please contact the Macmillan Corporate and Premium Sales Department at 1-800-221-7945, extension 5442, or write to specialmarkets@macmillan.com.

www.fsgbooks.com
www.twitter.com/fsgbooks • www.facebook.com/fsgbooks

1 3 5 7 9 10 8 6 4 2

For my mother
For Sonia
And for Mohan and Pia—always, always

Wholly unprepared, . . . we take the step into the afternoon of life; worse still, we take this step with the false assumption that our truths and ideals will serve as before. But we cannot live the afternoon of life according to the program of life's morning—for what was great in the morning will be little at evening, and what in the morning was true will at evening have become a lie. —Carl Jung

Contents

DOCTORED

Prologue: Storm

I am walking on a muddy path. The rain has ceased, and puddles are shimmering in the moonlight. I am wearing olive green Gap pants, beat-up Hugo Boss shoes, and an orange Patagonia Windbreaker. I am the picture of success.

I start to run. Trees and poles hurtle past me as head down, eyes fixed, I sprint down the trail. Wet leaves scrape against my face as I swat them away. Shadows oscillate. The wind is swirling like a loud yawn from heaven. I stumble on roots, but I keep on going.

Sleep has been hopeless. I haven't been able to nod off for more than a few hours at night, and sedatives leave me even groggier the following day. A strange feeling has taken hold of me, and it won't let go. "It isn't anger," I told Dr. Adams, my psychiatrist, "as much as butterflies in the stomach."

"Why the anxiety?"

"I don't know, but I am waking up with it and the workday hasn't even begun. How do I make it stop?"

My pants catch in nettled bramble. The cloth rips slightly as I struggle to free myself. I finally stop and gaze into the still blackness. A faint light glows in the distance, refracting through my spectacles into an array of crystals. In the damp weedy grass around me, crickets chirp in angry unison. A nearby branch quivers where a creature must have just departed. I begin to jog again. Misty droplets, heavier and more urgent, peck at my face until the sky opens up to release a downpour. I sprint home. You can speed up after an accident, but you never make up for lost time.

Introduction: Medicine at Midlife

> A certain amount of dissatisfaction may be inherent, even necessary,
> to the practice of medicine.
> —Abigail Zuger, *The New England Journal of Medicine*, 2004

When I look at my career at midlife, I realize that in many ways I have become the kind of doctor I never thought I'd be: impatient, occasionally indifferent, at times dismissive or paternalistic. Many of my colleagues are similarly struggling with the loss of their professional ideals. Of course, the relinquishment of one's ideals is standard fare in the midlife phase. In this period, fundamental questions about life often arise: What is its purpose? What is my ultimate aim? Depression and nostalgia can take hold as middle-aged adults struggle with responsibility, regret, and the nagging awareness that their lives are half over.

I used to think that my life would settle down when I got to this stage, but I was wrong. The insecurity and ambivalence of my youth have persisted, though in different forms. In my twenties, hamstrung by my passions, I yearned for consistency in my core beliefs. I obsessed about what I was going to do with my life. Those ruminations now seem like luxuries. The challenges I face now—supporting my family, navigating the precarious domains of job, marriage, and fatherhood while trying to maintain personal and professional integrity—seem so much bigger (if no less insoluble). As a young adult I believed that the world was accommodating, that it would indulge my ambitions. In middle age, reality overwhelms that faith. You see the constraints and corruption. Your desires give way to pragmatism. The conviction that anything is possible is essentially gone.

It occurs to me that my profession is in a sort of midlife crisis of its own. In the last four decades, doctors have lost the special status they used to enjoy. In the mid-twentieth century, at least, physicians were the pillars of any community. They made more money and earned more respect than just about any other type of professional. If you were smart and sincere and ambitious, the top of your class, there was nothing nobler or more rewarding that you could aspire to become. Doctors possessed special knowledge. They owned second homes. They were called upon in times of crisis. They were well-off, caring, and smart, the best kind of people you could know.

Today medicine is just another profession, and doctors have become like everybody else: insecure, discontented, and anxious about the future. In surveys, a majority of doctors express diminished enthusiasm for medicine and say they would discourage a friend or family member from entering the profession. In a 2008 survey of twelve thousand physicians, only 6 percent described their morale as positive. Eighty-four percent said their incomes were constant or decreasing. The majority said they did not have enough time to spend with patients because of paperwork, and nearly half said they planned to reduce the number of patients they would see in the next three years or stop practicing altogether. American doctors are suffering from a collective malaise. We strove, made sacrifices, and for what? For many, the job has become only that—a job.

Consider what a couple of doctors had to say on Sermo, the online community of more than 125,000 physicians:

> I wouldn't do it again, and it has nothing to do with the money. I get too little respect from patients, physician colleagues, and administrators, despite good clinical judgment, hard work, and compassion for my patients. Working up patients in the ER these days involves shotgunning multiple unnecessary tests (everybody gets a CT!) despite the fact that we know they don't need them, and being aware of the wastefulness of it all really sucks the love out of what you do. I feel like a pawn in a money-making game for hospital administrators. There are so many other ways I could have made my living and been more fulfilled. The sad part is we

chose medicine because we thought it was worthwhile and no-ble, but from what I have seen in my short career, it is a charade.

Another wrote:

I loved what I did, running an ICU. But I was on call 11 of every 14 days for more than 25 years. Over a third of my work weeks were 100 hours. I quit when I was 56 because my wife developed a terminal illness and I wanted to return all the lost hours I had promised her "when we retire." In my last year of practice I asked the billing department to collect all the actual money we had col-lected on one particularly long and difficult weekend on call . . . After overhead, I was actually paid $11.74/hour. Who would do that again? Fool that I am, I probably would, but my wife and I brought up our sons from an early age to be totally against the idea of medical school. They were clearly bright enough, with full academic scholarships. And while they respect physicians, they are not doctors. And I am glad they are not.

The discontent is alarming, but how did we get to this point? This book, chronicling my experiences in my first few years as a new doctor, is my attempt to answer this question.

———

A decade ago, the economist Julian Le Grand developed the idea that public policy is grounded in a conception of humans as "knights," "knaves," or "pawns." Knights are motivated by virtue. They want to make the world a better place. Knaves are selfish. They desire to extract as much as possible for themselves. Pawns are passive. They follow exter-nal rules and regulations rather than an internal code of conduct.

In a 2010 essay in *The Journal of the American Medical Association* (*JAMA*), Dr. Sachin H. Jain and Dr. Christine K. Cassel apply these concepts to medicine. Knights, they write, practice medicine to save and improve lives. The best thing government can do is to get out of their way and let them do their jobs. Knaves, on the other hand, put their financial well-being before their patients and often order tests for personal gain. Government needs to guard against their malfeasance.

Pawns are ruled by the environment in which they practice. The role of government is to incentivize them to do what is right. As Jain and Cassel write, "A society's view of human motivation influences whether it builds public policies that are permissive, punitive, or prescriptive."

The history of American medicine over the past half century can be interpreted through this lens. In the halcyon days of the mid-twentieth century, physicians were viewed as knights. They were among the most highly admired professionals, comparable to astronauts and Supreme Court justices. American medicine was also in a golden age. It was a period when life expectancy increased sharply (from sixty-five in 1940 to seventy-one years in 1970), aided by such triumphs of medical science as polio vaccination and heart-lung bypass. Doctors largely set their own hours and determined their own fees. Depictions of physicians in the media (*Marcus Welby, General Hospital*) were overwhelmingly positive, almost heroic. Doctors were able to trade on this cultural perception for an unusual degree of privilege and influence.

"Doctors were God," Harry Steinberg, the white-haired retired chairman of medicine at my hospital, Long Island Jewish Medical Center, told me. "They had the corner house in the neighborhood with the shingle out front. In the hospital they had their own private service. Everybody knew who you were. You walked around with a black bag, interns in tow. There was almost no regulation. We didn't have case managers telling us what to do. There weren't these interdisciplinary teams."

Suburban doctors in this period led a gentlemanly life. They'd go on rounds in the hospital in the early morning and then go to their offices—often attached to their homes—to see patients till noon. During their lunch break they might return to the hospital to eat in the doctors' lounge or to check on a sick patient, or they'd make a house call. In the afternoon they'd often go back to the hospital to check laboratory tests or X-rays or to meet with a patient's family, and get done with the bulk of their workday by 5:00 p.m. Evenings were spent at home with their families or at the social club or lodge. On Saturday nights they might have taken their wives out to dinner or even to the opera. In general, they weren't seeking patients. They desired respect and status in their communities. They worked hard but also lived with dignity and high-minded purpose.

Though he worked in a different country, my maternal grandfather led such a life. As a boy in India I used to watch him at work in the iodine-stained clinic on the ground floor of his palatial three-story flat in an upper-crusty neighborhood of New Delhi. Pitaji's clinic always smelled pungently of medicine, as did he. Through the drawing room window I'd spy him examining patients with boils or sepsis while lizards clung motionlessly to the limestone walls. He'd look so distinguished in his three-piece suit and spectacles, sitting cross-legged in an armchair beside books with titles such as *Diseases of Women* or *Treatment in General Practice*. His patients showed up at all hours, even during meals, and always without appointments: first come, first served. My grandmother functioned as his secretary and nurse. Grandchildren would be running around, playing cricket on the veranda, interrupting examinations, stealing his cystoscope or his magnifying glasses or the special otoscope with the brass earpiece. My grandfather was deeply proud of his knowledge. He fancied himself a mainstay of the community. He received fair compensation from those who could afford to pay and provided charity care to those who could not. Though it was a different time and place, this tableau matches well that of the American physician knight.

Indeed, American doctors at mid-century were generally content with their circumstances. They were prospering under the private fee-for-service model, in which patients were covering costs out of pocket or through fledgling private insurance programs, such as Blue Cross/Blue Shield. They could regulate fees based on a patient's ability to pay and look like benefactors. They were not subordinated to bureaucratic hierarchy. So when nationalized health insurance plans were proposed, doctors opposed them, perceiving an attempt to undermine income, autonomy, and, ultimately, patient care. They were afraid that the introduction of Medicare in 1965 would be the end of medicine as they knew it. It turned out they were right, but not in the way they imagined.

After Medicare was created as a social safety net for the elderly, doctors' salaries actually increased, as more people sought medical care. (Charity care also dwindled, as the federal government started to pick up the tab.) In 1940, in inflation-adjusted 2010 dollars, the mean income for American physicians was about $50,000. By 1970 it was close to $250,000, nearly six times the median household income. Doctors' purchasing power had never been greater.

But as doctors profited, they were no longer seen as knights. They were increasingly perceived as knaves bilking the system. Year after year, health care spending grew faster than the economy as a whole. Premiums for insurers like Blue Cross, whose reimbursement rates were determined by doctors, increased 25 to 50 percent annually. Meanwhile, reports of waste and fraud were rampant. A congressional investigation found that in 1974, surgeons performed 2.4 million unnecessary operations costing nearly $4 billion and resulting in nearly 12,000 deaths. In 1969 the president of the New Haven County Medical Society warned his colleagues "to quit strangling the goose that can lay those golden eggs.

"The temptation to get rich while the getting's good is powerful," he said. "A lot of our group have payments to make on their apartment house complexes [and] shopping centers . . . [But] you can't blame the average patient for thinking that we doctors are living much too high on the hog."

"It was a free-for-all," recalled a senior physician at my hospital who had worked through that era. "Before Medicare," he said, "doctors were not so focused on making money. Professional attainment still meant something. But if you call attention to this [change] you are considered a . . ." He struggled for the right word.

"Troublemaker?" I offered.

"Yes, a bad apple. There were so many unnecessary procedures. But all those doctors were board-certified," he said disappointedly. "Who was I to tell them what to do?"

If doctors were mismanaging their patients' care, someone else would have to manage that care for them. Beginning in 1970, health maintenance organizations (a term coined by Paul Ellwood, Jr., a physician and an aide to President Richard M. Nixon) were championed to promote a new kind of health care delivery built around price controls and fixed payments. Unlike with Medicare or private insurance, doctors themselves would be held responsible for excess spending. There were other novel mechanisms for curtailing health outlays, including greater cost sharing by patients and insurer review of the necessity of medical services. The Health Maintenance Organization Act in 1973 supplied grants to start new HMOs to provide such "managed care" and required businesses with more than twenty-five workers to offer an HMO option, if available, thus ushering in a new era of health care financing.

The transition from knighthood to knavery had major consequences for doctors. In 1973 fewer than 15 percent of physicians reported any doubts that they had made the right career choice. By 1981 half said they would not recommend the practice of medicine as highly as they would have a decade earlier. Public opinion of doctors shifted distinctly downward, too. Doctors were no longer unquestioningly exalted. There were journalistic and media critiques of the medical profession. On television, for example, physicians were portrayed as more human—flawed or vulnerable (*M*A*S*H**, *St. Elsewhere*) or professionally and personally fallible (*ER*).

As managed care grew (by the early 2000s, 95 percent of insured workers were in some sort of managed care plan), physicians' confidence plummeted further. In 2001, 58 percent of about two thousand physicians questioned said their enthusiasm for medicine had gone down in the previous five years, and 87 percent said their overall morale had declined during that time. More recent surveys have shown that 30 to 40 percent of practicing physicians would not choose to enter the medical profession if they were deciding on a career again, and an even higher percentage would not encourage their children to pursue a medical career.

There are many reasons for this disillusionment besides managed care. An unintended consequence of progress is that physicians increasingly say they have inadequate time to spend with patients. Medical advances have transformed once terminal diseases—cancer, AIDS, congestive heart failure—into complex chronic conditions that must be managed long term. Physicians also have more diagnostic and treatment options and must provide a growing array of screenings and other preventative services. In a study of sixty-seven hundred patients in twelve metropolitan areas, researchers found that the medical care for a host of ailments, including diabetes, alcoholism, and pneumonia, met national guidelines only slightly more than half the time. A paper published a decade ago in the *American Journal of Public Health* estimated that it would take over four hours a day for a general internist to provide just the preventative care—scheduling mammograms, arranging screening colonoscopies, and so on—that is currently recommended for an average-size panel of adult patients (this on top of the regular workday managing acute problems and emergencies). "The amount of time required is overwhelming," the authors wrote. If anything, the problem has worsened since then.

However, the dissatisfaction probably would not have reached such a fever pitch if salaries under managed care had kept pace with doctors' expectations. But they have not. In 1970 the average inflation-adjusted income of general practitioners was $185,000. In 2010 it was $161,000, despite a near doubling of the number of patients that doctors see per day. While patients today are undoubtedly paying more for medical care, less and less of that money is actually going to the people who provide the care. According to an article in the journal *Academic Medicine*, the return on educational investment for primary care physicians, adjusted for differences in number of hours worked, is just under $6 per hour, as compared with $11 for lawyers. As in the rest of America, there is serious income inequality in the medical profession. Some doctors, especially procedure-based specialists, are probably paid too much. Others, such as primary care physicians, are not paid enough. (Yet almost every doctor feels the world owes them more for what they've been through.) Doctors today are working harder and faster to maintain income, even as staff salaries and cost-of-living expenses continue to rise and medical school debt approaches $200,000. Some have resorted to selling herbal supplements and vitamins out of their offices to make up for decreasing revenues. Others are limiting their practices to patients who can pay out of pocket without insurance company discounting. Private practices today are like cars on a hill with the parking brakes on. When you look at them, you don't realize how much force is being applied just to maintain stasis.

"I am very dissatisfied," a doctor wrote online. "My father was a family physician . . . We discussed how maybe the practice of medicine should be reserved for the independently wealthy or a religious order. Seriously, I fear that these pressures will drive suicide and mental disease sky-high within our group of colleagues, who for the most part went into medicine due to the size of their hearts with minimal consideration on the impact of the size of their wallets. We all thought we would be comfortable and be able to pay our bills. All I have to say is, thank God my wife works."

The time crunch and reimbursement cuts are only a small part of doctors' woes, however. Other factors include a labyrinthine payer bureaucracy (American doctors spend almost an hour on average each day, and $83,000 per year—four times their Canadian counterparts—dealing with the paperwork of insurance companies); fear of lawsuits; runaway malpractice liability premiums; and finally, the loss of professional autonomy that has led many physicians to view themselves as pawns in a battle between insurers and the government. A doctor lamented on medscape.com: "The public policy forces acting upon us are pushing us into being technicians on an assembly line with less and less time to relate to our patients as people and sometimes hindering us from even giving the best technical care. But we can only work so hard and so long, and if our patients aren't willing to pay for better time and attention, then we have to change with the times."

The growing discontent has serious consequences for patients. One is a looming shortage of doctors, especially in primary care, which has the lowest reimbursement of all the medical specialties and probably has the most dissatisfied practitioners. Try getting a timely appointment with your family doctor. In some parts of the country today, it is next to impossible. A report published by the Association of American Medical Colleges projected a shortage of as many as 150,000 physicians by 2025. Aging baby boomers are starting to become patients just as aging baby boomer physicians are getting ready to retire. The nation is going to need new doctors, especially geriatricians and other primary care physicians, to care for these patients. But interest in primary care is at an all-time low.

Perhaps the most serious downside, however, is that unhappy doctors make for unhappy patients. Patients today are increasingly disenchanted with a medical system that is often indifferent to their needs. There has always been a divide between patients and doctors, given the disparity in power inherent in their relationship, but this chasm is widening because of time constraints, malpractice fears, decreasing income, and other stresses that have sapped the motivation of doctors to connect with their patients.

People used to talk about "my doctor." Of course, you had other doctors as the need arose, but you had one doctor you could call your own, and when you were sick, that doctor would be at your bedside. The archetype of a loyal, empathic family physician persisted in our culture for decades.

Today care is widely dispersed. In a given year, Medicare patients see on average two different primary care physicians and five specialists working in four separate practices. For many of us, it is rare to find a primary physician who can remember us from visit to visit, let alone come to know us in depth or with any meaning or relevancy. Many primary care physicians are no longer able to care for their patients who have been admitted to the hospital, relying instead on hospitalists devoted to inpatient care. It has become prohibitively inefficient for primary care physicians to leave the office for several hours—to drive to a hospital, examine a patient, check laboratory tests and vital signs, talk to a nurse, and write orders and a note—for just one or two patients. The economic calculus is such that if they did this on a regular basis, they wouldn't have enough revenue to pay their staff, their rent, and their malpractice insurance. The upshot is that the doctor who knows a patient best is often uninvolved in her care when she is hospitalized. This contributes to the poor coordination and wanton consultation that are so common in hospitals today. "Years ago you had one or two doctors," a hospitalized patient told me. "Now you've got so many people coming in it's hard to know who's who."

Not long ago I took care of a woman with an abdominal mass who had been transferred to my hospital for a preoperative evaluation. No one knew exactly what the mass represented or even whether she had had a biopsy—including the physician at my hospital who had accepted the transfer. The paperwork from the other hospital was a mess, incomplete; no one could make any sense of it. And the doctor we reached at the transferring hospital knew next to nothing about the patient. I told my patient that there were some things we needed to figure out before sending her to the operating room. "Like what?" she asked.

"Like what is this mass," I answered. "Is it cancer? Has it spread?"

"Do you know if it has?"

"I don't, ma'am. I'm just meeting you for the first time."

Tears filled her eyes. "No one knows what is going on," she said, and she was right. I was eventually able to tell her it was a benign mass, but not before she had been tortured by worry for two days. It is hard to imagine such a thing happening in the era of "my doctor."

Insensitivity in patient-doctor interactions has become almost normal. I once took care of a patient who developed kidney failure after receiving contrast dye for a CT scan. On rounds he recalled for me a conversation he'd had with his nephrologist about whether his kidney function was going to get better. "The doctor said, 'What do you mean?'"

my patient told me. "I said, 'Are my kidneys going to come back?' He said, 'How long have you been on dialysis?' I said, 'A few days.' And then he thought for a moment and said, 'Nah, I don't think they're going to come back.'" My patient broke into sobs. "'Nah, I don't think they're going to come back.' That's what he said to me. Just like that."

Of course, doctors are not the only professionals who are unhappy today. Many professions, including law and teaching, have become constrained by corporate structures, resulting in loss of autonomy, status, and respect. But as the sociologist Paul Starr writes, for most of the twentieth century, medicine was "the heroic exception that sustained the waning tradition of independent professionalism." It is an exception whose time has expired.

―――――

This book is not only about the midlife crisis in American medicine, but also about my own struggles as a middle-aged doctor, husband, and father to find equilibrium in my life and my practice. In my book *Intern* I describe the formative years of my medical training at a New York City hospital. *Doctored* is the further story of an education, about the loss of ideals and about midlife corrections and solutions. In fractal geometry, there is the concept of self-similarity, in which component parts resemble the whole. As in a coastline, reiteration of patterns occurs at progressively smaller scales. The premise of this book is that much can be learned about how to heal American medicine, forty years old in its modern incarnation, in a midlife portrait of one of its practitioners.

Everything that appears on these pages actually happened. However, most names and identifying details have been changed to preserve confidentiality; in some places, time has been compressed or the order of events has been changed for the sake of narrative cohesion; and in rare cases I have used composite sketches to better represent my experience. Dialogue is usually based on notes taken at the time, though some has been reconstructed from my memory.

The practice of medicine today is as fraught as it's ever been, and the doctor-patient relationship is in serious trouble. One of my goals in writing this book is to understand why. These are not trivial problems. How they are resolved will in no small part determine the future of health care in this country.

PART I

AMBITION

ONE

Awakening

A young doctor means a new graveyard.   —German proverb

I had been pedaling furiously for nearly a decade—on a stationary bicycle. Medical school, internship, residency, and fellowship: my education seemed as if it would never end. So it was with no small measure of relief that in the late spring of 2004 I accepted a position as an attending cardiologist at Long Island Jewish Medical Center in New Hyde Park, New York. This was the last step in a long and grueling journey. After medical school I'd completed three years of hospital instruction in general internal medicine to earn the privilege to practice independently. After finishing this internship and residency, I'd elected to do a fellowship: three more years of study in cardiac diseases to further specialize. Now, with the fellowship concluded, I'd become an attending physician, the senior level of the hospital hierarchy, with ultimate responsibility for patients and junior doctors. Nineteen years after starting college and a few months shy of my thirty-sixth birthday, I finally had my first real job. The complexities of academic medical training had long since worn thin. I was ready to simplify, consolidate, and perhaps even reap some rewards for all those sleepless nights.

Cardiology was a natural career choice. I had trained as a physicist before going to medical school, and the heart, with its complex rhythms and oscillations, appealed to my predilection for patterns and logic. Heart disease was also no stranger in my family. Both my grandfathers had died of myocardial infarctions—one in his forties, ten years before I was born—so I had grown up with an awe of the heart as the executioner of men in the prime of their lives. Plus, the heart, with its symbolic meanings, had always occupied a special place in my (and the broader cultural) imagination. Take heart! Have a heart! He wears his heart on his sleeve.

Of course, I was nervous. Every new doctor should be. Cardiologists specialize in emergencies. The culture is fast-paced, pressured. I was going to have to learn to become quick and decisive in precarious situations. By nature I was slow and deliberate, and I had never felt comfortable acting on instinct—not exactly adaptive in a cardiac care unit where people can drop dead on you at any moment. In neuroscience there is the concept of the reflex arc, in which a threatening stimulus can effect a response without passing through the conscious brain—for example, when you see the taillight flash red on the car speeding in front of you and your foot automatically moves to the brake pedal. I was afraid that as a cardiologist I would now have to follow a similar reflex arc.

"Well begun is half done," my father reminded me with his usual Aesopian wisdom. Dad possessed the annoying certitude that there were no more life lessons to be learned in this world, that whatever was worth knowing our forebears had already taught us. Traditional and moralistic, he liberally quoted proverbs and scriptures even if he didn't always live by them. But when you think in axioms and parables, when the collective wisdom of the world can be distilled into the concentrated tonic of a few sayings, then you feel as though you have all the answers.

He had always wanted me to become a doctor—one trained at Stanford University, no less. That, he believed, would be the pinnacle of professional attainment. My family immigrated to the United States in 1977, when I was eight, to advance my father's career as a plant geneticist, but in America my father never achieved the kind of success he felt he deserved—denied, he believed, by a racist university tenure system, which forced him to take postdoctoral positions with no long-term stability and left him embittered and in a constant state of conflict with professional colleagues. In medicine, my father explained, I would not be plagued with such insecurity.

One reason for my father's struggles was that he always seemed to do things the wrong way. When I told him the mnemonic I had learned in school to remember the colors of the spectrum, he said: "Roy G. Biv? Oh, you mean Vibgyor!" He'd mow the lawn at night, waking the neighbors. He'd bring up controversial subjects like Sikh separatism or Kashmiri violence at low-key social gatherings. He'd trim our nails with a Gillette razor blade, twisting our fingers painfully so they wouldn't get lacerated. As long as the nails got cut, it didn't matter to my father how much we protested. That sort of encapsulated his personality: disciplined, unsentimental, focused solely on the task at hand.

My mother affectionately called him *poottha*, "awkward." She accepted his idiosyncrasies with a kind of bemused resignation, as if they had been written in the stars. The eldest daughter of a wealthy New Delhi physician, she abided her station as the working wife of a discontented plant geneticist as though it had been ordained, just part of the deal of an arranged marriage, and she resolved to make the most of it. She didn't believe in talk or analysis or drama, only in putting your best foot forward and grinding ahead, accepting your circumstances with dignity and grace. Yet for all her equanimity, she still regarded medicine as the hammer that would break her children out of the middle-class mold my father had set. She often told us she wanted her children to become doctors so people would stand when we walked into a room.

My apprehensions about my new job were only slightly mitigated by the fact that my older brother, Rajiv, an interventional cardiologist who performed invasive procedures, was already working at the same hospital. Rajiv was my parents' firstborn, their pride. They had always favored him, and Rajiv demanded it, too. He knew the privileges of being the elder son in a traditional Indian family and guarded them closely, like a trust fund. Like most brothers close in age, we were fiercely competitive growing up, evenly matched at most things (Ping-Pong, chess, tennis), our rivalrous parity enforced by the unspoken fear that if one of us pulled away, we'd lose the other's companionship. One sphere in which we were undoubtedly unequal was social relationships, however. Rajiv had the kind of gregarious and easygoing personality that I had always desired but somehow never could develop. The only time we had worked together professionally was during my internship at New York Hospital in Manhattan, where as a star senior cardiology fellow he unwittingly reminded me of my incompetence again and again. Toward the end of my own cardiology fellowship at NYU, he had invited me to apply to LIJ and had used his considerable influence to get me a job. Now he was in a position to guide me through another, perhaps more challenging apprenticeship.

At Long Island Jewish I would work as a cardiologist with a specialization in congestive heart failure. This was no small task: heart failure is the common final pathway for a host of cardiac diseases, including heart attacks, acute valve disorders, viral infections of the cardiac muscle, etc. There are many challenges in caring for these patients. They have multiple comorbid illnesses, such as diabetes and emphysema. Their symptoms—for instance, shortness of breath—are often nonspecific. They frequently have poor health literacy or cognitive impairment or are socially isolated because of their chronic disease. Despite these difficulties, I chose to specialize in heart failure because I wanted to develop close relationships with critically ill patients and provide long-term care, unlike my brother, who almost exclusively performs procedures and knows his patients mostly for the duration of an operation. I also wanted to be in a specialty where I would not have to perform surgical interventions. I'd never been especially good with my hands. Growing up, Rajiv had been the tinkerer and I had been the thinker. Of course, I knew this decision was going to involve a certain degree of monetary sacrifice. Heart failure is a money loser for most hospitals, which make most of their revenue from lucrative procedures like stents (wire mesh cylinders used to open blockages in the coronary arteries that feed the heart) and pacemakers, or hip replacements. In the American system doctors are paid much less for exercising their judgment than their fingers.

———

Dawn in July, a few weeks after starting my new job. Sirens puncture the early-morning stillness. I open my eyes. Twilight leaks through the window blinds, dissolving the gloom into tiny grains of black. I remain motionless, savoring the void. My wife, Sonia, is still sleeping—sleeping for two. I peer at the hazy sonogram framed on the windowsill. It is faded from the sunlight that beats on it daily, betraying nothing of the complications of the past few months.

I get up quietly and tiptoe to the bathroom. In the mirror I notice I've developed a touch of gray. A bracing splash, some bloody nicks, a suitable tie, and I am outside. It is a bright day, nearly cloudless, the skyline marred only by the steam drizzling out of a tower in the distance. I pull out of my building and drive north, past empty playgrounds and cracked brownstones and apartment complexes stacked like Lego blocks. Street sweepers are out in force, ravenously whirling over the grime and debris. I turn onto the FDR Drive. A few joggers are out on that lonely stretch of waterfront. A couple of miles on, I enter the blue-green expanse of the Triborough Bridge. Pigeons flutter off the ramparts. Across the shimmering East River, skyscrapers in Midtown are arrayed like an irregular bed of nails. I press on the gas pedal. The brilliant day is pulling me forward.

I was asked during job interviews how I planned to create a heart failure program. I replied that if you provided good care and vigilant monitoring and were responsive to patients' needs, community physicians would refer their patients. I had no idea if this was actually true; but it sounded good, and I got the job. I promised to decrease lengths of stay, improve hospital performance measures, improve the discharge process, decrease readmissions, install a computerized database, enroll patients in clinical trials, write emergency room protocols, and start an intravenous infusion clinic. Eventually I wanted to hire a nurse practitioner, a dietitian, a social worker, and a physical therapist. But I had accomplished none of these things as I drove to work that July morning.

It was a few minutes past seven-thirty when I arrived at the hospital, and I was late for morning report. I pulled into the attending physicians' lot and parked between two cars whose license plates read "BEAN DOC" and "GAS MD." At the sliding glass doors leading into the lobby, two patients in teal hospital gowns were leaning on their IV poles, sucking hungrily on cigarettes. I skipped down a concrete stairwell to the basement. The corridors were deserted, save for a tardy first-year fellow racing ahead of me.

When I walked into the conference room, a fellow was presenting a case from overnight. About a dozen fellows and a half-dozen faculty members were there. The fellows rotated each month through the various cardiac subspecialties: electrophysiology (which focuses on arrhythmias, or heart rhythm disturbances), echocardiography (cardiac ultrasound), nuclear stress testing (which uses radioactive tracers to noninvasively detect coronary disease in hearts under stress from exercise or certain drugs), cardiac catheterization (Rajiv's specialty), heart failure, the general consultative service, and the cardiac care unit (where the most critically ill patients of any subspecialty usually ended up). As faculty members we were responsible for teaching the fellows: scrubbing in with them on procedures, going on rounds with them, and instructing them over discussions at morning report or noon seminar. In the conference room, Rajiv and two of his interventional colleagues were sitting together, arms folded, legs crossed, in purple scrubs, like some sort of academic tribunal. My brother looked at me sharply, glanced at a phantom wristwatch, and winked. I quietly took a seat in the back.

The fellow was trying to explain his management of a critically ill patient the previous night. "The patient's pulmonary artery saturation was in the mid-forties, so I ended up putting him on some dobutamine and gave him a little fluid back," the fellow said. "He started putting out some urine, and his blood pressure went up. Over the next twelve hours, his oxygenation improved dramatically."

Dr. Morrison, one of the interventional cardiologists, demanded to know why the fellow had given the patient intravenous fluid.

"At that point his central venous pressure was two," the fellow said defensively, describing a state of dehydration. "His pulmonary artery diastolic pressure was six, and his wedge pressure was like eight."

"And you're sure the transducer was zeroed and level?" Morrison pressed him. "We see this a lot with the residents. They look up at the monitor and quote a pressure, but it's just garbage."

The fellow hesitated. "When we first put in the catheter, the wedge pressure was in the thirties—"

"Well, see, that's what I'm saying," Morrison interjected, as if the fellow had just made his point. "This guy wasn't dehydrated! He was in florid heart failure. This is a textbook case of acute heart failure, from the frothy sputum to the missed myocardial infarction."

"Anyway, good case," the chief fellow said, trying to move things along.

"What this patient really needs is a doctor," Dr. Morrison added caustically.

"As opposed to a plumber like us?" Rajiv shot back, coming to the fellow's defense.

"Exactly," Morrison replied, laughing. (Interventional cardiologists who relieve coronary obstructions with stents are often disparagingly referred to as plumbers.)

Looking around the room, I reminded myself how lucky I was to be working at a teaching hospital where residents and fellows would be making rounds on my patients and assisting me on cases. LIJ is one of the largest teaching facilities on Long Island, sitting on fifty acres on the Queens–Long Island border, housing nearly eight hundred beds, and employing seven hundred physicians on its full-time faculty. The evidence shows that patients treated for several common medical disorders, including heart failure, heart attack, and stroke, fare better at major teaching hospitals and have better overall survival. One reason may simply be redundancy: residents and fellows may be annoying when you're reciting the details of your fainting episode for the third time in the middle of the night—"So tell me, did you pass out before or after you hit the floor?"—but so many pairs of eyes on each patient mean things don't get overlooked. Eighty percent of medical diagnoses can probably be made on the basis of a patient's history, and the more people asking, the more likely doctors are to get it right. Another factor is the sheer number of patients treated at the average teaching hospital. Patient mortality tends to drop as doctors get more experience. Would you rather have angioplasty performed by a cardiologist who does two hundred a year—or twenty?

Though I'd been hired to start a heart failure program, I'd been informed that for the first year or so I'd also be assuming frequent responsibility for the cardiac care unit (CCU), where I'd be treating not only patients with heart failure but also those with other, more general cardiac problems (myocardial infarctions, arrhythmias, etc.) to help me build up my practice. So after morning report, I headed up to the CCU, where I was substituting for Dr. Vaccaro, the director, who was on vacation that week. Fifty years ago there were only about a hundred "special care" coronary units in the United States. Since then there has been a veritable hailstorm of cardiac advances, including implantable pacemakers, prosthetic heart valves, coronary bypass surgery, and heart transplantation. Today most hospitals with more than a hundred beds have a cardiac care unit.

Chiming alarms reminiscent of a video arcade greeted me when I arrived. The CCU was a refurbished unit with gleaming tile and a distinctly modern feel. The faintly pleasant odors of disinfectant and talcum powder wafted through the corridors. Nurses were weaving in and out of rooms, attending to their patients. Families were loitering in the hallways or sitting at bedsides, keeping vigil. At the front desk an old woman gruffly answered the phone. "CCU, Eva, may I help?"

As I joined the team for rounds that morning, the bleary-eyed post-call fellow was signing out to Ethan, the CCU day fellow. Ethan was a short Jewish guy with glasses that were too big for his face, spiky gelled hair, and a geeky hyperexcitability. Like most fellows, he was eager to make a good impression. He was constantly toeing that fine line between being assertive and kissing ass.

The postcall fellow was telling Ethan about a cardiac arrest from the previous night. "You're doing things, and you're doing them because you've got to do them, but you're thinking, Why the hell am I doing this?" he said, shaking his head in resignation.

"Sometimes it's out of your hands," Ethan said sympathetically.

"I told the daughter I was going to go down swinging—"

"It wouldn't have mattered," Ethan interrupted. "It was a finger in the dike. That patient was destined to die, and that's all there is to it."

The postcall fellow nodded appreciatively. After he departed, Ethan turned to me and said matter-of-factly, "We got lucky, Dr. Jauhar. One transfer patient didn't show up, one patient the private attending decided he didn't want the consult, and one patient died."

The team of doctors in the CCU consisted of Ethan, three residents, and three interns, including Paul, a nerdy East Asian who was supposed to quickly present overnight admissions and leave the hospital by 10:00 a.m. to meet the latest work-hour regulations. As an intern I would never have been allowed to leave the hospital before completing all my responsibilities for the day, but times had changed. All week I'd constantly been checking my team's work, pushing them to do what they were supposed to be doing, nothing extra. Just getting the trainees to do what was expected of them was hard enough. Everyone was casually dressed—oxford shirts but no ties—not what I remembered from my own residency. Huddled around the rolling chart rack in the hallway, we stopped outside the first room.

"Jerry Simons is a forty-nine-year-old man with a history of drug abuse who was admitted to another hospital on Friday after doing cocaine," Paul narrated. He chuckled before continuing. "He was sitting in his kitchen having dinner when he broke into a sweat. His wife noticed his shirt was drenched, so she got him a towel, and then he changed his clothes, but they got drenched, too—"

"You can just say he was diaphoretic," I interrupted.

Paul nodded. "He started having chest pain. He described it as a burning, or rather squeezing, pressure, not really sharp, though it had a pins-and-needle—"

"Just show me the electrocardiogram," I said, trying to hurry him along.

Paul pulled it out of his coat pocket. An electrocardiogram, or EKG, measures the electrical signals coming from the heart. On this one were ST segment elevations, a serious abnormality, indicating an acute attack, or infarction, of the inferior wall of the heart.

"Do you see a Wellens sign?" Ethan asked me, referring to an esoteric EKG finding. I shook my head. The residents stared blankly.

Paul continued, taking no notice of Ethan's ass-kissing: "So in the ER he reported shortness of breath and light-headedness. He had ST elevations but didn't spill any cardiac enzymes," the latter indicating irreversible damage to the heart muscle.

"All right, let's go see him," I announced.

Before we walked into the room, Paul quickly added: "By the way, he doesn't want to talk about his drug use. He already told me he wasn't going to stop."

Mr. Simons appeared to be sleeping when we got to the bedside. He was a thin black man with curly gray hair and a grizzled face. The sheets were off, and his gown was pulled up. There was a bloody patch on his right groin where a cardiac catheter had been inserted. He opened his eyes slowly when I started to speak. I introduced the team and asked him how he was feeling.

"I just swallowed some pills," he said flatly.

"Oh, did you swallow them the wrong way?" I asked.

He gazed indifferently at the roomful of doctors. "Before you came in, the nurse gave me my pills, so when you said how you doing, I said I swallowed my pills." He threw a blanket over his exposed leg. "That's all."

I applied my stethoscope to his chest. His heart was racing, perhaps a sign of drug withdrawal. I explained to him that we would normally start him on a beta-blocker to slow down the rate, but the medication had a potentially harmful interaction with cocaine. Was he planning on using again?

"All you cats love throwing that word 'cocaine' around," he said, his voice rising. "I don't want to hear that word again."

"Look, I don't know whether you regularly use drugs or not," I said, my jaw tightening. "I just want to know about the future, so I can decide how best to treat you." Moral reform was not my objective. Getting him on the right medications was.

"You don't know nothing about me," he said angrily.

"I know that cocaine is addictive."

"I'm not addicted!"

"Then why don't you quit?"

"I did! Yesterday."

I told him he was going to have to follow up as an outpatient and undergo at least two negative drug screens before I would prescribe him a beta-blocker. "You have to do something," I lectured him. "You're on the path to self-destruction."

He stared at me tensely for a few moments. "I know I've got to quit," he said quietly. "I tell myself I'm going to stop, and then the pipe just appears in my hand. It's gone in thirty seconds, and I don't even know what I've done."

The cast of patients in the CCU that morning was similar to Mr. Simons: sick, indigent, on a slow journey to dignity. Arthur Batista in room 6 weighed over 350 pounds. His body resembled a collection of interconnecting spheres: soccer balls for thighs, a bag of tennis balls around his waist, and a beach ball for a rump. He had an unsightly growth of facial hair, a thick, almost absent neck, and the rancid odor of someone who has too much body surface to wash. His heart was functioning at less than half capacity. He was standing with one foot on a banana peel, as a nurse put it.

When we walked into his room, he was lying on his side, trying to generate enough momentum to stand up. There was a large stain on his bed, which explained the musty smell. "Man, this is just crazy!" he cried, pulling on a fluid-filled plastic line. "I'm all tangled up. I have to get up and take a piss!"

Four of us helped him to his feet, rotating an IV pole twice around his body to untangle the line. While we remained assembled around him, he peed into a plastic urinal. Just that bit of exertion made him winded, and he plunked down into a sofa chair.

"How is your breathing today, Arthur?" I asked pleasantly.

"My breathing's fine," he said, even though he was panting. He pointed up at the monitor. "I don't think I even need the oxygen anymore, but they're going by the numbers up there." He picked up his face mask. "This thing is broken. I need you to call the respiratory therapist and get me a new one." I told him we would.

A nurse's aide barreled in to check his blood sugar. In one seemingly continuous motion, she prepared the lancet, swabbed his fingertip with an alcohol pad, pricked the finger, coaxed a droplet of blood onto a card, and inserted the card into a glucometer. Then she turned and walked out.

"What's the number?" he roared as she slipped away. "They always walk out before they give you the number!"

The howl brought his nurse in. "What's the matter, Arthur? You okay?"

"I'm fine!"

"He was all tangled up," I explained.

"I had to stand up to pee, okay! To do that, I have to take off the oxygen."

"Not a problem," the nurse said calmly. "Just ring the buzzer."

"That's what I did! Nobody comes." Scowling, he turned to me. "The first day they're fine, but after that they ignore you." He surveyed the group of doctors standing around him. "You guys just keep throwing pills at me. One doctor says one thing; another doctor comes in and says, 'No, you got a problem with your kidney.' Now, which one is it, guys? You should get your stories straight."

I told him that our role as the cardiac team was to focus on his heart condition. Different doctors were managing his kidney problems.

To judge from his groan of frustration, such division of labor did not sit well with him. (There was an inverse relationship, I'd discovered, between patient satisfaction and the number of doctors coming and going through their hospital rooms.) He placed his hand on his scrotum, edematous from the fluid overload of heart failure. "My nuts are starting to go down," he announced. "So when can I go home, Doc?" I told him that he would likely have to go to a rehabilitation facility first.

"Rehab? What the hell for?"

"To get you stronger."

"But I'm fine! This doctor"—he pointed at Paul, the intern—"whatever his name is, Chao—"

"Cheung," Paul corrected him.

"Whatever. He was telling me something else."

"Well, I'm running the show here," I said.

"Then let me go home."

I hesitated. "I'm just covering for the week. I'll have to speak with Dr. Vaccaro."

Exasperated, he shook his head. "Well, if I had known that, I would've just invited you to sit down and play cards!"

The most tragic case in the unit was Delmore Richardson, a forty-eight-year-old man who had collapsed three weeks prior after coming home from a dinner party. His wife had recounted the event for me. "He walked into the bedroom, but then he kind of stumbled and held on to the doorjamb," she said. "I watched him fall backward. He bashed his head on the floor. First, I thought he was having a seizure. He kind of went *awwgh*." She made a deep, guttural sound. "I yelled for my brother. He came downstairs and started doing chest compressions. I tried to breathe for him. His mouth was open, but every now and then he'd go *awwgh*." She stopped, overwhelmed by the memory. "We called 911. They shocked him twice. It was pandemonium. There were so many people working on him, I got pushed into the kitchen." When I asked where her children were, her lips quivered. "Unfortunately, their bedrooms are right off the living room, so they walked in on it. They saw the whole thing."

Mr. Richardson had clearly suffered significant brain damage because he had been out so long. That morning, on rounds, his arms and feet were splayed rigidly outward in a position called decorticate posturing, a sign of severe neurological injury. Air bags, inflating and deflating to prevent blood clots, were wrapped around his immobile legs. A bottle of medicated fluid, hanging on a metal pole, dripped into his vein. A plastic tube in his rectum was draining pond green diarrhea, which was decanting into a bag, solids on bottom, clear liquid on top. His head rested on a towel, which caught secretions from the breathing tube taped to his chin. The ventilator recorded the respiratory rate: machine: 11; patient: 11. He wasn't breathing on his own at all.

A nurse slipped a thin plastic catheter down the breathing tube. With her thumb covering a hole in the vacuum line, she suctioned out thick yellow secretions, which pooled into a bucket. With her help, I hauled him onto his side and listened to his back, which was slippery with ointment. On his tailbone was gauze dressing, which I pulled aside to inspect the bedsore underneath, a pink crater about the size of a small saucer but less than half the depth. Inside it were tiny black flecks, perhaps dead tissue. I picked up his swollen arm. An allergy band was eating into the wrist, leaving a deep furrow. I let the arm go and it dropped with a thud. I used a pen to stroke up on the soles of his feet, unwittingly peeling up dead skin. Both big toes went up, a primitive reflex seen in newborns, a sign in adults of neurological devastation.

Emma, his wife, had been keeping vigil for three weeks, spending most days (and some nights) on a small flower-patterned couch by the window. She was a pretty, muscular woman who, despite the tragedy unfolding before her, still managed to maintain a brave front embellished with lip gloss and eye shadow. "He is going to pull out of this," she had told me adamantly. "I have hope he is going to walk out of here."

But by then there was virtually no hope for any sort of meaningful recovery. His blood pressure was starting to fluctuate. He had unexplained fevers. He was entering the downward spiral of the terminally ill, where competing problems grow in significance, where a solution to one problem causes another.

"Did he ever express any wishes about intensive care?" I'd asked her. "About being on a respirator or life support?"

"No, we never had that conversation," she answered, shaking her head sadly. "We joked once about a close friend who was sick, how we wanted to keep him alive, but that was just joking."

Without a do-not-resuscitate (DNR) order, we were going to have to try to revive him if he had another cardiac arrest, a possibility we all dreaded. "I know you want him to get better," I told his wife that morning on rounds, trying to convince her again to sign the paper. "It is only human to want to see improvement, but the chances of him going back to the way he was are basically nil." It sounded harsh, even to me, and I was sorry I had to say it. I reminded her that he would soon require a tracheostomy, during which a breathing tube would have to be inserted externally into an incision in his throat just below his Adam's apple. We couldn't leave him with an oral breathing tube much longer without inviting serious complications.

"Well, I am not agreeing to that right now," she said, waving off the suggestion. "And I am not going to make him DNR either. He just needs more time. All these medicines and antibiotics are making it harder for him to breathe—"

"If we stop the antibiotics, he will die," I said sharply. "And he has been off sedatives for at least a week."

"It's only been six days," she replied. "Last Sunday it looked like he was ready to go home with me."

I had encountered such resistance many times in my career, when loved ones see only what they want to see. As in those cases, it was obvious to me that our efforts here were futile and that they were only going to make him end his life more miserably. "So you would want us to do CPR if his heart stopped?" I said, no longer trying to hide my disapproval.

"Yes, of course," she replied, as though it were the most obvious thing in the world. "Give him the best possible chance to wake up, even if it's just to say goodbye."

A nurse was seated in front of a computer monitor outside the room. "She would never do this if she had to pay for it," she snapped when I came outside. And though I cringed at her flippancy, she was probably right. Some of the wastefulness in hospitals, I'd learned, especially in intensive care units, is driven by families unable to let go. I sat down to pen a note while the team moved on. The nurse turned to me. "She doesn't understand his brain is mush and where he is going from here. We keep telling her, but she just looks at you with this blank stare." She turned back to the monitor and clicked the mouse. "God, I hate buying used cars!" she cried.

Rounds lasted about three hours. By the time we were finished, there was a plan in place for all the patients. After leaving the unit to go to my office, I stopped by the cath lab to add a patient's name to the board. The cath suite, like most procedure rooms at the hospital, was shiny and new. Fluorescent lights created a zigzagging stream on the polished tile.

Rajiv was sitting at a console in one of the control rooms, finishing up a report. Tapping on the keyboard, he spoke fawningly on the phone with a referring physician. "No, sir . . . yes, sir . . . okay, *ji* . . . yes, boss . . . no, Plavix is for six months only, boss . . . okay, boss . . . okay, boss . . . thank you, boss . . . thanks, boss."

No doctor I'd ever met took the business of medicine more seriously than Rajiv. He was the ultimate rainmaker, taking referrals 24-7 from his vast network of physician friends. He viewed medicine on Long Island as a ruthless competition in which only the most adaptable and socially savvy would survive. He boasted that his success derived from the three A's: availability, accessibility, and affability (virtues, he claimed, that he'd learned from private practitioners and applied to his salaried hospital practice). He always carried his beeper, even when he wasn't on call. People could (and would) reach him at all hours. He even attended the notoriously dull Indian doctor parties. "I'm a prostitute," he once crowed. "I'm not ashamed; hell, I bring Vandana. I make her socialize with all the Indian ladies." His wife had smiled, a knowing, resigned smile. "I ask him, 'Just this weekend, can we have family time? Do we have to go to another party?' But he says it's good for business."

After Rajiv hung up the phone, I gave him a quick update on his patients in the CCU. Ms. Wink had acute kidney injury, so we had decided to do a pharmacological stress test instead of a catheterization with potentially kidney-toxic dye. Mr. Lawner was whacked-out and noncompliant, plus, his family was loopy, so I had decided he should get no further testing. Ms. Sankar was a new patient with unstable angina. She needed to be catheterized that afternoon . . .

Before I could finish, Rajiv put his arm around me in an unexpected show of affection and gave the back of my neck a hard squeeze. "It's great seeing you every day," he said, beaming as I winced in pain. "I still can't believe you're here."

———

That afternoon, on 7-North, the cardiac ward, I quickly saw three CCU outliers, patients who had been stabilized and no longer required intensive monitoring. When I sat down to write my notes, it was almost 3:30 p.m. How limited our interactions with patients, I thought. We see them for a few minutes, then pen a quick summary and leave directions for the nurses to follow. To whom are we speaking in these inky chart drizzles? Doctors, patients, a phantom lawyer ("I spoke with the patient at length, but he is still refusing . . .")? Or perhaps we are just talking to ourselves, regurgitating the patient's history to create a tidy narrative. The audience shifts, patient to patient, note to note, even sentence to sentence.

At four o'clock, while I was finishing up my last note, Ethan, the CCU fellow, paged me. "Mr. Richardson just dropped his pressure," he said nervously about the brain-damaged patient in the CCU. "I tried going up on the Levophed and the Neo-Sinephrine, but it didn't work. When I turned on vasopressin, his pressure dropped even more."

I thought for a moment. This was the kind of situation I'd feared most as an attending, when I had to respond almost reflexively. (And how hard should I try to save a severely brain-damaged patient anyway?) All the medications Ethan had mentioned had half-lives, so it was hard to know how to interpret the results. "I would back off on the vaso," I said carefully. "Just start some dobutamine at 2.5 micrograms per kilogram per minute. I'll be there in a couple of minutes. Did you call the wife?"

"I got through to her a few minutes ago," he replied. "I told her to come right away."

When I arrived back in the CCU, the code had already begun. A group of doctors and nurses were at the bedside. The rhythm on the monitor was ventricular fibrillation, random electrical oscillations. An intern was doing chest compressions. Saline was running wide open through an IV. Defibrillator pads adhered to Richardson's hairy chest. His body jerked up and down with every administered shock. Because his heart had effectively stopped, his lungs had filled up with pink, frothy liquid, mostly blood plasma, like beaten-up Jell-O, which came up through his breathing tube. The compressions sent the nurses scrambling for face masks and yellow gowns to protect themselves from the red spray.

"This is a conspiracy to prevent me from getting my afternoon coffee," quipped a doctor who had shown up to help. I chuckled at the wry shoptalk.

After a couple of adrenaline injections, Mr. Richardson regained a pulse; but it immediately started to die down, and within a few minutes it disappeared. It seemed his body had finally given up. The sequence continued: shocks, chest compressions, and drugs. He got four doses of adrenaline at 1 milligram each, then 5 milligrams, then 10, but the pulse did not return. He received several ampoules of sodium bicarbonate. By then he was blue in the face, a sickening color, like an old hematoma. We continued CPR while I called for an echo machine, which takes ultrasound pictures of the heart. "Let's take a quick peek before we call it," I said. When the machine was wheeled in, I pulled the window shades closed and applied the ultrasound probe to his chest. The heart was in standstill, hazy clots filling the ventricles. I pressed a button to take a picture. The room was quiet as I pronounced him dead.

Gowns and masks were stuffed into a trash bin, and people started filing out of the room. Then a strange thing happened. My gloved fingertips, soaked with blood on his pulseless groin, started to vibrate. Wait, I ordered the group.

In the Bible, Lazarus is raised from the dead by Jesus. In medicine, Lazarus is the patient who, believed dead, spontaneously starts to circulate blood.

About forty cases of the Lazarus phenomenon, a number that experts believe is too small to be valid, have been reported in the medical literature. (I have seen at least three cases in my own career.) Though most patients died soon after the event, in eight cases they left the hospital, neurological functions intact. The cases share a kind of morbidity: A man, eighty, is pronounced dead after thirty minutes of CPR. His doctor showers and returns five minutes later to find his patient has a pulse. A man, eighty-four, goes into cardiac arrest while biking. After fifteen minutes of CPR he is pronounced dead and taken to a mortuary, where attendants see him breathing. A woman, sixty-eight, suffers a heart attack and goes into prolonged cardiac arrest. Removed from her ventilator, she is taken to a separate room, where about twenty minutes later a nurse notes she is breathing and moving under the sheet. She is discharged from the hospital and dies three months later in her sleep.

Why are certain deaths "reversible"? The phenomenon remains a mystery. Some have speculated that cessation of CPR decreases pressure in the chest cavity, allowing blood to return to the heart. In 1993 a doctor described the Lazarus phenomenon in a seventy-five-year-old man with a lung hemorrhage. "How [increased blood return] would stimulate the completely quiescent myocardium . . . is not readily apparent," he wrote. "There had been no electrical cardiac activity . . . for several minutes at the time the efforts were terminated. This situation spontaneously reversed."

There is even a kind of Lazarus phenomenon that has been described in brain-dead patients who make spontaneous movements after they are disconnected from ventilators. Patients have been observed to develop goose bumps on their arms and trunk, raise and flex their arms rapidly, and display complex finger movements. A doctor described one patient raising his arms off the bed and extending his elbows, as if performing a benediction, and another crossing his hands in front of his neck, as if grasping for his breathing tube. These movements sometimes occur despite no measurable blood flow to the brain. Some doctors speculate they are generated in the spinal cord.

However, as with most Lazarus patients, Mr. Richardson's awakening was short-lived. After about five minutes his pulse disappeared, and despite a few more doses of adrenaline, it never returned. He was pronounced dead a second time after about ten minutes.

I found his wife sitting in the waiting room. She looked up when I walked in. "Is it over?" she asked.

"Yes," I replied.

"Did he die?"

I put my arm around her. She began to cry. "I'm sorry," I said.

As I drove home that night around eight, Long Island Sound was pitch-black, apart from the glimmering reflection of light poles. Fat rain droplets, like little eggs, started to splatter on my windshield, smearing with each sway of the wipers. In the distance the fractured skyline of the city stood out like shards of glass. Though I was physically exhausted, my mind was filled with the heady, mysterious events of the day. What had restarted Mr. Richardson's heart? Was it the delayed action of adrenaline? Was it the bicarbonate? Was it something else?

In Harlem the roads shimmered shiny black. Red taillights winked at me through the watery haze. Police sirens were sounding out loudly. On 116th Street, dented low riders slinked by, windows open, music blaring. My headlights caught a lonely figure under the elevated train tracks.

I called Sonia to tell her that I was almost home. "How did Lamaze go?" I asked. Regrettably, I had missed it again this week. There was silence. "Honey?" I heard sobs.

"We need to talk," she finally said, composing herself. "Dr. Edwards just called. She thinks the baby is in danger. She says I need a C-section before she goes on vacation next week."

TWO

Odd Conceptions

> Patients' decisions about their care must be paramount, as long as
> those decisions are in keeping with ethical practice and do not lead to
> demands for inappropriate care.   —Physicians' charter

Sonia and I'd had a hard time conceiving, but not because of a lack of
diligence. We tried everything: ovulation sensors, Kokopelli figurines,
yoga, meditation, Clomid, Pergonal, intrauterine injections, in vitro fer-
tilization (IVF), even mystical appeals to a Hindu guru (who confidently
predicted we would have two boys). Nothing worked. The failures left
us feeling tense and frustrated.

In early 2003, at the midway point of my fellowship and shortly after
our third unsuccessful attempt at IVF, we went on vacation to the Caribbean island of Anguilla. We both needed a break. We had been trying to get pregnant for over two years—Sonia was now thirty-two, and I
was thirty-four—and we were quietly panicking that our efforts had become futile. One afternoon shortly after we arrived, I went for a walk
alone on the sun-swept beach, where I met a shirtless loafer named
Clement Clemons. He was tall and handsome, with brown dreadlocks
emanating from his red bandanna and a quiet, dignified island air. We
got to talking, and by and by he invited me to his "tavern," a tourist attraction just up the road, where he said we could get "happy together."
With Sonia relaxing by the pool at the hotel, I accepted his proposition.
After hopping about two hundred yards on the scorching white sand, we
arrived at the back entrance to a bamboo shack, where a group of Amer-

icans were lounging on cheap rattan furniture, taking hits from a water pipe. Tiny lamps dangling from wooden beams bathed the room in a chocolaty orange. I sat down, and almost immediately the rim of a water bong was sealed around my lips and thick white smoke was gurgling through a purple curlicue shaft. The giggling tourists egged me on. It was a scene right out of the dorms at Berkeley.

Soon towering speakers were piping out joyful Dead tunes, and I was tripping heavily in a hallucinatory mix of speed and calm. Out on the deck, I gazed at a stunning palm-fringed tableau. It felt as if I were in a movie, a contrived visual narrative of an unsuspecting traveler stoned to oblivion in a foreign land. My mind was moving randomly through an array of interconnecting circles. Why is there space? How did it arise? Why are there jeans and tile floors and chairs of different material? So much we don't understand!

Clement joined me on the terrace. His bandanna gave the illusion of streaming the colors of the rainbow. "This is the strongest shit I've ever smoked," I told him, feeling dizzy. He just laughed.

The late-afternoon sun cast long shadows across the wooden deck. The sky was painted in swirls of pastel mixed with bubbly streaks of white. It reminded me of springtime in Berkeley, and thus of Lisa, my college girlfriend. What had happened to her? Where was she now? The last time we'd spoken was before I got married, when she recalled the scooter rides in the Berkeley Hills in those carefree early days. So strange that I didn't still think about her every day: those brown curls and milky white skin; the raffish grin. At one time all paths of thought had converged on her. I used to obsess about her, her disease—lupus— and the miscarriages doctors predicted she'd have. I remembered that birthday eve when my father asked me, "Don't you want children?" and my anguish for her gave way to my own desires. In the end, I abandoned her because I didn't have the courage to cope with her illness. I gave her up to avoid the terrible fate of being without her.

I suddenly became aware that Clement was talking to me. "Why you so serious?" he said.

I shook my head and continued to gaze at the beach.

"Somethin' is botherin' you," he said. I glanced at him. Fervidness was radiating from his dirty yellow sclera. I mentioned the problems that Sonia and I were having.

"You are injurin' yourself," he intoned. "And you are hurtin' her, too."

I nodded, staring at the turquoise water.

"Don't worry," he said. "You will have a boy."

I turned to him. His face was vibrating. "A boy?" I said.

He nodded confidently. "A son."

"How do you know?"

"Because I am a Rastafarian."

"What does that mean?"

"It means I believe in me, and I believe in you, too."

That night I told Sonia about Clement's prediction. She seemed pleased. Though neither of us really cared whether we had a boy or a girl, Sonia, having grown up in a family of girls—two sisters, mostly female cousins—had been hoping for at least one boy. Later at the hotel, lying awake in bed, I told myself that if I ever had a child, I would be a different kind of father from my own dad, who had been too busy with his professional struggles to develop friendships with his children. He did a passable job—acceptable in that era—and we all ended up just fine. But he didn't elevate to the highest ranks of parenting. He used coarse tools, like guilt, to foster the behavior he desired. I wanted to be a father with influence—in a good way—over his kids, unlike Dad, who had been too preoccupied with his own problems to garner that authority.

Just as Clement prophesied, Sonia did get pregnant a few months after we returned from Anguilla, and all signs pointed to our having a boy. The first sign presented itself at the beginning of the second trimester, when a homeless man, stooped and stinking and clutching a Bible, turned to us as we were walking along Seventy-seventh Street and shouted, "It's a boy!" A week later, as we were riding on an elevator in our building, a four-year-old boy pointed at Sonia's gravid belly and whispered something to his mother. After we stepped out at the ground floor, Sonia tapped me on the shoulder. "Did he just say . . ." She hesitated.

I nodded.

"What?" she demanded.

"He said, 'It's a boy,'" I replied.

Pleasantly spooked, she sank into a soft couch in the lobby and laughed. That is what she had heard, too.

Life, for the most part, was good. The tension of getting pregnant had evaporated. I was near the end of my fellowship and starting to interview for jobs (and was looking forward to finally achieving some financial security). Sonia herself was finishing her internal medicine residency at Lenox Hill Hospital on the Upper East Side and was mulling an offer to become chief resident for a year. After the stress of the previous two years, we couldn't have asked for a smoother patch.

But then, midway through the second trimester, Sonia developed a complication of pregnancy that required us to choose between two surgical treatments: one was standard; the other, which we selected, was more novel and appealing. Two weeks later we found ourselves at the Ambulatory Surgery center at Roosevelt Hospital. Sonia was lying on a narrow gurney in a room with four or five other patients. An intake nurse went over her medications, allergies, and medical history. When I told her that Sonia was eighteen weeks pregnant, she switched pens to mark down this fact in bright red ink. Soon Sonia was hooked up to a fetal monitor, which traced a normal heartbeat on pink graph paper.

A few minutes before the operation was scheduled to begin, a physician's assistant came up and demanded that Sonia sign a consent form for the standard surgery we did not want. When she refused, he said the operation was going to be canceled. Perplexed, I demanded to speak with our surgeon, Dr. Levinson.

"We were told this was our decision," I cried when he showed up a half hour later.

"I'm just learning about this now," Levinson replied calmly. He was a stocky Jewish surgeon in his late forties with an impressive professional record, including stints at the National Institutes of Health, that belied his awkward, slightly vacant air. He explained that the anesthesiologist, with whom he exclusively worked on such cases, had decided the procedure we had chosen wasn't safe because he couldn't ensure that our baby would get sufficient oxygen during surgery, an assessment that Sonia and I, as doctors, as well as our obstetrician, Dr. Edwards, with whom we had consulted, did not agree with. "I know you're upset—"

"Upset? I'm furious! We thought everything was a go, and now you're telling me this?"

"Everything I told you was correct from the way I understood it when we spoke—"

"Then tell me you're going to do the operation. We'll sign anything you want. These asshole anesthesiologists always raise objections. They don't know the patient or the situation."

"I understand—"

"I don't need understanding!" I shouted. "All I want to talk about is how we can make this happen." I was infuriated, not only by the precarious position in which we now found ourselves but also because I was sure that the unfounded fear of a lawsuit was at least partially driving the anesthesiologist's decision. Nearly half of all anesthesiologists, and almost 100 percent of physicians in high-risk specialties such as neurosurgery, cardiology, and obstetrics, will face a medical malpractice claim at some point in their careers. Malpractice litigation is often the most stressful experience in a doctor's professional life. Most doctors do not discuss it with colleagues or even with family members; it is a hidden shame. And though I might have sympathized with the anesthesiologist if I'd been on the other side of the doctor-patient dyad, none of this mattered to me as my pregnant wife lay on a gurney. Dr. Levinson was silent. "I'll go to the head of the hospital if I have to," I threatened, but I could tell from his expression that there was nothing more he was going to be able to do.

Trembling with anger, I left the room and went back to Sonia in the preoperative waiting area. I sat down beside her and stroked her hand. Looking at my face, she started to cry.

As the hours wore on, I continued to press our case. I demanded explanations. I asked for second opinions. When I requested that the anesthesiologist, a handsome Italian fellow with a bushy mustache, more business executive than doctor—and we, it seemed to me, more like job applicants than patients—recuse himself, he snapped that he did not want to talk in "lawyerly" language. He was acting almost like a conscientious objector, but I wasn't sure what he was objecting to. Which moral principle was he defending? First do no harm? Professional integrity? A paternalistic duty to protect his patient from a mistake? Or were his considerations being driven by more knavish concerns? My father-in-law, also a doctor, tried to negotiate. No one would budge.

So, finally, we said no. I wasn't going to let Sonia be pressured into an operation she did not want. At six o'clock, after waiting in the hospital for almost eleven hours, we went home to think about what to do.

Our case illustrates a basic conflict in modern American medicine. A patient's right to self-determination is the prevailing ethic, but in reality doctors routinely place limits on it. For example, when a patient's demand clashes with a doctor's moral convictions, ethicists have argued that doctors can deny treatment. Gynecologists can refuse to perform abortions because of moral or religious beliefs. Physicians in intensive care units often withhold treatments they deem futile, especially for terminal illnesses (as I tried to do with Delmore Richardson, the brain-damaged patient in the CCU).

But conscientious objection is a relatively rare impetus for denying treatment. A more common situation is one in which a patient's request conflicts with what a doctor believes to be good medical practice (and thus exposes the doctor to a possible charge of malpractice). In such cases the objection is over professional, not moral, integrity, though obviously moral questions are raised. In a doctor-patient dispute, who has the right to make the final call? Should doctors just do a patient's bidding? We talk about a patient's right to refuse treatment. But what about the right to demand it?

After I had started working at LIJ, a few months past this incident, I took care of a middle-aged man who had been admitted to the hospital with fever and shortness of breath. The man, Eric, was in his early forties, thin but toned, with colorful tattoos and a pallid countenance. A chest X-ray in the emergency room showed fluid in his lungs, but initially we did not know why it was there. An echocardiogram provided the answer. On one of his heart valves was an infected mass of tissue, a vegetation, flapping around wildly like a flag in the breeze. It had severely damaged the valve, resulting in congestive heart failure.

Heart infections, caused by bacteria entering the bloodstream, can usually be treated with intravenous antibiotics; surgery is reserved for only the most complicated cases. In Eric's case, a CT scan of the head showed several small bleeding sites, probably caused by parts of the vegetation breaking off and lodging in his brain. Surgeons decided that the valve needed to be replaced to prevent further injury.

A consulting neurologist recommended an MRI (magnetic resonance imaging) before surgery to make sure the infection had not caused any brain aneurysms that could rupture and bleed in the operating room, causing a stroke. When the scan showed no aneurysms, the neurologist asked for a cerebral angiogram to exclude even tiny aneurysms that the MRI might have missed. Though fairly routine, angiograms in rare cases can cause strokes because a catheter is threaded into the arteries that supply blood to the brain. Eric decided that although he wanted the surgery, he did not want this test.

"You know what I think," he said to me. "I think they're just throwing everything at this, and maybe they'll find something, and then what? They got an MRI, and they're still not satisfied!"

I explained that the doctors were being cautious.

"Hey, I'll sit here with antibiotics going into me, no problem," he replied. "But doing a procedure that could cause a stroke? That's getting a little scary."

I pulled out my stethoscope so I could listen to his lungs. What if he refused the angiogram? he asked, leaning forward. Couldn't he have the operation anyway?

I told him that the surgeon would probably not operate without the angiogram, a hunch confirmed the following day.

"But what if I sign a paper accepting the risk?"

The outlines of a memory started to form in my mind. "I doubt that's going to change anyone's mind," I said. I told him that if he felt strongly enough, I could arrange for him to be transferred to another hospital.

He did not want to do that. "Oh well, it is what it is," he said, looking resigned. "They're going to get what they want. It's a losing battle."

Though I agreed with the neurologist that an angiogram was needed before surgery, given the risks of even a tiny aneurysm bleeding during the operation, I felt uncomfortable about forcing Eric to have it. He had made it clear that he wanted to proceed with surgery without delay or additional testing. He was willing to accept the risks of this approach. But his doctors refused to honor this request.

How should such disputes be resolved? It isn't always clear. In 1991 a Minnesota court ruled that the family of Helga Wanglie, an eighty-six-year-old woman in a coma, had the right to demand intensive medical treatment for her, even though her physicians wanted to stop life support because they believed it was futile. In that judgment, patient (or surrogate) autonomy trumped professional integrity. However, in most cases of medical futility, doctors have been allowed to exercise conscientious objection.

In part because of my own experience with Sonia and the baby, I have come to believe that doctors should deny treatment requests judiciously—and rarely. A surgeon might understandably refuse to operate on someone whose religious beliefs proscribe blood transfusions on the ground that he would not want to be forced into medical malpractice. But in cases with reasonable differences of opinion, in which the competing risks are at least debatable, it seems unfair and unwise to me to deny a patient's choice. (If patient autonomy means anything, then patients have the right to make bad decisions, too.) Was Sonia's anesthesiologist being virtuous or knavish? I'm still not sure. Professional integrity can indeed be a double-edged sword.

In the end, we flew to the world-famous Cleveland Clinic, where a young surgeon agreed to perform the operation we wanted. The brushed marble columns and labyrinthine corridors of the hospital lent an air of competence and credibility that we were desperately seeking. At our first appointment, a nurse with a Midwestern twang and a midwife's manner came out to greet us. She shuttled Sonia through a quick triage and obtained her medical history. The surgeon came by around 11:00 a.m. I told him about our experience in New York. "If the patient says no, you have to listen to the patient," he said kindly. "You have to be suspicious when a doctor is so dogmatic."

We slept fitfully in the hospital the night before the surgery. Nurses came by every few hours to check blood pressure and vital signs. In the middle of the night, Sonia wanted me to take her for a walk. We wandered down mostly empty corridors to the chapel, a long and narrow chamber with stained-glass windows and a prominently displayed leather prayer book. Pro forma, I whispered a prayer. I hadn't prayed in years, but at this point I would have done anything to stack the odds in our favor. After wandering into an adjoining room, I came back to find that Sonia was gone. I went outside, but I could not find her. I called her name, but she did not respond. I was about to leave when I saw her praying quietly in a pew at the front of the chapel. In the prayer book she had written: "Dear Lord, lead me the way to a complete cure."

The chief of high-risk obstetrics came by in the morning, while I was in the cafeteria getting breakfast. With a fellow, she quickly performed a fetal ultrasound. She asked Sonia if she wanted to know the gender of the baby. Sonia said she preferred to wait until I returned. She asked the obstetrician to come back later to talk to both of us.

Back in the room, we waited nervously for a transporter. We still didn't know the sex, but Sonia assured me: "We're going to be all right. Our baby boy is my guardian angel, so don't worry."

At the surgical unit I was handed a pager and told that someone would call me when the operation was over. About an hour later, as I was pacing nervously in the family waiting area, the device buzzed. I hurried over to the front desk, where a nurse in blue scrubs and bonnet told me that the procedure had gone smoothly and that Sonia was already in the postanesthesia care unit. I rushed to her bedside. Though she was still groggy, she gripped my hand tightly, obviously elated. While waiting for her to fully wake up, I went to a hospital phone and paged the obstetrician. I introduced myself and asked her if she could tell me the sex of the baby. "You don't want to wait for your wife?" she teased. I told her that Sonia was in recovery and that I would inform her later.

"It's a bit early to tell for sure," she hedged, "and we didn't get the best pictures, but it looks like you're having a girl!" A girl? Stunned, I said nothing, so sure had both of us been that it was a boy.

I thanked the obstetrician and wandered into a gift shop, where I bought a tiny figurine. In the recovery unit I gave it to Sonia. "Why pink?" she asked, still dazed. I told her what the obstetrician had told me. Smiling, Sonia said, "She is going to be my beauty, my tennis partner."

In fact, the chief of obstetrics at the Cleveland Clinic turned out to have been wrong. We were actually having a boy, which was confirmed by an ultrasound two weeks later, after we had returned to New York. "Are you absolutely sure?" I pressed Mary, our flower-child, friendship-braceleted sonographer. I mentioned what we had been told in Cleveland.

"Oh, I'm pretty sure," she said, "but let me check again." She twisted the probe, trying to get clearer images. "Yes, see that? It's definitely a boy." She took a picture, which we put into a metal frame on the windowsill in our bedroom. I couldn't help but laugh. The little boy in the elevator, the homeless guy on Seventy-seventh Street, and Clement, the Rastafarian, had all gotten it right. But not the chief of maternal-fetal medicine at the world-famous Cleveland Clinic with the aid of ultrasound!

We became addicted to monitoring our baby. Just for kicks, we'd sneak into the echo lab at NYU, where Sonia would lie on an exam table and I, a senior cardiology fellow, would gently press the cardiac ultrasound probe to her belly. Her eyes would twinkle, and I would smile, too, quietly overjoyed at the melding of my personal and professional lives. We spent hours watching a video I made of our baby throwing up his arms, startled. We couldn't pull ourselves away from him.

Then, in the thirty-fourth week of the pregnancy, with everything finally going smoothly, Dr. Edwards called Sonia at home and told her to schedule a caesarean section. She said she wanted to avoid any risk of further complications.

"I told her that I needed to discuss it with you," Sonia said when I returned from the hospital that night, just after I had started my new job at LIJ. "It was like she wanted me to agree with her right on the spot because she said for the umpteenth time, totally well-meaning, I'm sure, 'I don't want you to feel antagonistic, I'm on your side,' and in the most polite way possible I was, like, 'Dr. E, I'm just asking questions.' I'm sure she's used to her patients just agreeing with her. Anyway, she's available to see us tomorrow. She wants us to decide this week."

We met at her office on East Seventy-second Street the following afternoon. Sitting across a desk from us, she explained her reasoning. The baby was mature. He should be delivered under the most controlled circumstances. Waiting until the baby was full-term would only invite further problems. I mentioned data I'd found nervously scouring the obstetrical literature suggesting that a vaginal delivery might be safer because it caused fewer alterations in maternal blood flow. But Edwards replied that this evidence was based on small studies that were not clearly applicable to our case. One problem with clinical research is that the profile of subjects rarely matches that of the patient in front of you. In the end, she made a convincing case and we reluctantly acquiesced, though it obviously wasn't what we had hoped for.

The weekend before the scheduled C-section, I took my first call as a new attending. It was a busy weekend. I had to see patients at both LIJ and its sister institution, North Shore University Hospital, in Manhasset. On Saturday morning an elderly woman actually had an acute stroke while I was making my rounds. When I first visited her, she was speaking normally, asking to go home. Twenty minutes later a nurse paged me to say the patient was insensate, aphasic, and frothing at the mouth. She was totally mute when I ran upstairs to see her, her mouth drooping to one side, a look of alarm on her face. After rushing to the nurses' station, I directed an intern to order an emergent CT scan of the brain and to page the neurologist on call. Unbelievably, the intern refused, saying that she was at the end of a twenty-four-hour shift and was going home. In fact, her insubordination had been legislated in 2003, the year prior, in rigid work-hour restrictions limiting residents to twenty-four hours on call, with three additional hours to hand off their patients. The caps were supposed to improve the learning environment by providing medical trainees with more opportunities to rest, but they seemed to have had the opposite effect, encouraging a kind of shiftwork mentality. Having done my own residency without strict work-hour limits, I believed that you had to see a patient's illness through its course—observe the arc—to get a grip on the dynamics of the disease. I worried that the current crop of interns, mandated to leave the hospital after a long shift, was missing out on valuable lessons and was learning a mentality of moderation that is incompatible with the highest ideals of doctoring. As a resident I would never have insisted on leaving the hospital during an emergency involving one of my patients. However, I didn't argue with this intern, and I ordered the scan and made the calls myself. The CT scan confirmed what I suspected, a huge stroke involving the left middle cerebral artery, and the patient was transferred immediately to the intensive care unit under the care of the neurology team.

All weekend Sonia and I had second thoughts about the scheduled C-section, so we kept calling each other to talk it over and be reassured. At lunchtime, sitting in a conference room with a pile of four hundred EKGs and a turkey sandwich, I found myself stupidly calling the Cleveland Clinic, anonymously asking the obstetrician on call whether a two-week preterm delivery could result in any long-term impairment. At the computer in my office on Sunday afternoon, I obsessively looked up obstetrical abstracts on outcomes for elective C-section. But despite the anxiety, in the end we decided to stick with Dr. Edwards's plan. On Sunday night, after I got home, amid the new crib we were still assembling and the new changing table and the boxes of diapers and baby paraphernalia, we quickly packed our bags to go to the hospital the following morning.

The operating room on the afternoon of Monday, August 9, 2004, was reassuringly abuzz: alongside Dr. Edwards were two obstetrics fellows, an anesthesiologist, a neonatologist, several nurses, and, of course, Sonia, swathed in blankets, staring anxiously up at the ceiling. Her father had told Edwards that delivering the baby before two-thirty in the afternoon would be especially auspicious, according to a Hindu guru he'd consulted, so it was a silly race against the clock, which added a sense of tension that we didn't really need but was vaguely exciting nevertheless.

It took about thirty minutes for the anesthetic to reach the level of Sonia's belly. The wisecracking anesthesiologist kept testing her thighs and abdomen with a sharp needle, leaving tiny bleeding marks on her skin. When the anesthetic finally reached the level of her chest, the operation could begin.

I stole peeks into the operating field. Tiny yellow globules of fat glistened as the Bovie knife broke the skin. Soon amniotic fluid spilled forth, to be slurped up quickly by a suction catheter. I watched as Edwards tugged on the uterus with red-soaked gauze and a metal retractor. Blood spilled on the white tile floor. Then suddenly our baby was out, tethered by an umbilical cord. A couple of gentle taps and he started wailing; the room broke into applause.

I swooned, and for a moment I thought I was going to black out. Weeks, months, years of worry melted away in an instant. Edwards clamped the umbilical cord and cut it, and then started sewing up the uterus with big black stitches. Our newborn was placed into the arms of a neonatology fellow and rushed over to a warming table. Someone called out to me to take a picture. I breathed an enormous sigh of relief—fertility injections, the trip to Anguilla, the reluctant anesthesiologist, and the Cleveland Clinic all flashed in rapid succession through my mind—and another one the following day when Sonia went to the postpartum unit to breast-feed our healthy baby boy.

THREE

Learning Curve

The art of medicine, like that of war, is murderous and conjectural.

—Voltaire

On Friday, three days after the delivery and about six weeks after I'd started working at LIJ, I pulled up on the cobblestone roundabout behind New York Hospital to pick up Sonia and our newborn baby, Mohan, and drive them to Sonia's parents' home in Edison, New Jersey. Meanwhile, my parents and my sister, Suneeta, went to Long Island to stay with my brother. My parents stayed with Rajiv whenever they visited New York, a deference they naturally extended to their greatest asset and biggest investment.

On Sunday morning, after I had spent a long night helping Sonia with feeding and diaper changing, Rajiv phoned me in a panic. My father had been having episodes of numbness and tingling in his left arm (along with similar but milder symptoms on the right). Rajiv was worried they were transient ischemic attacks (TIAs), or ministrokes. He said he was taking my father to LIJ to be evaluated.

"Stroke?" I said dubiously. "With bilateral symptoms? Come on, what kind of nerve distribution causes bilateral—"

"Don't be academic about this!" Rajiv snapped, cutting me off. "Let's let the experts figure out what's going on."

He called me a couple of hours later. Caroline Davenport, the neurologist on call, had seen my father in the emergency room. Suspecting a TIA, she'd sent him for a CT scan of the brain, which was normal.

Since early strokes don't always manifest on a CT scan, she had ordered an MRI of the head and brain stem, which also revealed nothing unusual. Despite the normal studies, she had decided to admit my father for observation and started him on blood thinners.

I jumped into my car and sped to the hospital. It was a calm and clear day, a stark contrast with the maelstrom that had been unleashed in my chest. Though I doubted anything was seriously wrong with my father—I'd seen him only a couple of days earlier, and he hadn't mentioned any symptoms to me—I still felt afraid. Dad wasn't supposed to get sick. It was the one thing as children we were told to fear the most. I raced across the George Washington Bridge. The Hudson River was shimmering like a pool of mercury. Near La Guardia Airport, I got stuck in a traffic jam, honking my horn in desperation to get it moving while airplanes drifted precariously low overhead. By the time I reached the hospital it was already past noon, two and a half hours after I had departed.

I found my father in a semiprivate room on the seventh floor. His eyes were darting, and he had a strangely disconnected look, which I attributed to anxiety. Rajiv and my mother were there, too, sitting quietly, now looking bored. A medicated drip hanging on a pole was connected to my father's arm. Rajiv informed me that Dad's blood pressure was elevated, so doctors had given him lisinopril, the same drug that we had advised him to start several years earlier but that he had declined. We now took turns assailing him over how irresponsible he had been. He offered no defense.

The reason my father had refused to take lisinopril (or any other drug Rajiv and I had suggested) was that he no longer trusted medicines to keep him well. Six years earlier, when I was in my final year of medical school, he had started having headaches that were probably triggered by job stress but that over the course of several months became chronic. Initially he took over-the-counter medications like Tylenol and aspirin, but with little relief. Then, at the urging of doctors, he moved on to prescription drugs: Flexeril, Fiorinal, Imitrex, amitriptyline, Paxil, and finally, prednisone. During that period he was seen by an array of specialists: three internists, two neurologists, two rheumatologists, an anesthesiologist, and an ophthalmologist. No one could tell him what was wrong. Then one day, totally fed up, my father stopped all his medications. Two weeks later, his headaches were gone.

"It was the medicine that was causing the headaches," he concluded incredulously (and probably correctly). And though he'd grown up in a culture in which doctors commanded tremendous respect, he'd been loath to listen to physicians ever since.

The following day in the hospital, my father got an echocardiogram to see if there was a blood clot in his heart that could have partially dis-. lodged and landed up in his brain. There was not. He also got a trans-esophageal echo, in which an ultrasound camera was passed via a stiff tube into his mouth, down his throat (numbed with anesthetic), and into his esophagus to get close-up views of his heart. Apart from showing a mildly leaky aortic valve, probably a result of hypertension, it, too, was unremarkable. Again Rajiv and I got on his case about his blood pressure. "Do you want to end up with a stroke?" I blared. (Admittedly, I derived some pleasure from the scolding after a lifetime of his preaching.) "You won't be able to work."

"I'd rather be dead," my father replied quietly.

Over the next couple of days, my father underwent a battery of further tests: carotid ultrasound, transcranial Doppler, lower-extremity Doppler, and chest CT. It seemed a bit excessive to me, but I said nothing. The studies were normal. Since he was symptom-free with no speech or other neurological deficits, Dr. Davenport decided to observe him for one more day and then send him home. We hardly saw her during the hospital stay. Even when she did show up, she spent no more than a couple of minutes with my father and then rushed off. On the day of discharge, my father was given prescriptions for four medications—lisinopril, aspirin, Lipitor (a cholesterol-lowering drug), and Aggrenox (a blood thinner used to prevent strokes)—and was told to follow up with a neurologist once he got back home. Grateful for the reprieve, and appreciative of the efforts of his doctors, he said he had learned a lesson and pledged to take his medications regularly and his health more seriously.

Three days later, when I was back at work, my sister, Suneeta, called me from Rajiv's house, where she and my parents were still staying. Dad's symptoms had returned, worse than ever. He now had virtually no sensation remaining in his left arm.

"But he's had all the tests," I said skeptically. "Let me talk to him."

Suneeta was hysterical. "He says he's having a stroke!" she shrieked.

"He says he can't feel his arm!" The strength she struggled to show as the baby girl in a traditional Indian family often devolved into anger or panic under pressure. In the background I could hear my mother yelling out in alarm, as though my father were falling down.

"It is happening," my father announced when he finally got on the phone.

"What?" I demanded.

"I don't know, but I think I am dying."

He had never sounded so frightened to me. I told him I would call an ambulance, but he insisted that Vandana, Rajiv's wife, drive him immediately to the hospital.

About an hour later I heard "LIJ, code stroke to the emergency room" over the intercom. Racing downstairs—even though I was running, I still didn't believe anything could be seriously wrong—I arrived to find Robert Holman, Dr. Davenport's portly associate, evaluating my father on a stretcher with a neurology resident and a rather severe-looking Filipino nurse. My father was whisked away for another head CT before I could even talk to him. When it revealed nothing new, preparations were made for a repeat MRI. As my father lay there among shouting drunks and screaming children, appearing about as miserable as I'd ever seen him, a nurse took me aside. "Don't know if I should mention this, Dr. Jauhar, but I've noticed your father's symptoms get worse when he tilts his head," she said. She'd had him do certain maneuvers, like touching his chin to his sternum, that reproduced his symptoms exactly. I went over to his stretcher and had him repeat the motions. "That's it," my father said, dipping his chin down unnaturally. "Now I cannot feel my arm."

I found Dr. Holman in the radiology room, reviewing the head CT for any subtle abnormalities. When I informed him of the nurse's findings, he walked over to my father and, apparently examining him for the first time because the doctor looked so surprised, had him perform the exercises again. Sure enough, the numbness was reproducible, suggesting that my father only had a pinched cervical nerve, a relatively benign condition. Appearing chastened, Holman said the MRI was now probably unnecessary but advised my father to have it anyway (with the imaging extending into the neck) to eliminate any residual uncertainty. It confirmed what the nurse had suspected: a pinched nerve.

My father was given a prescription for a neck brace and sent home from the ER. I decided not to tell him too much about the final diagnosis. I didn't want to ratify his distrust of doctors, and I wanted to maintain a little fear in him so he'd take his blood pressure medication. The following day, he and my mother flew back home to Fargo, North Dakota, where he was then working as a plant geneticist.

A few weeks later I was having breakfast with Tom Antoni, a newly hired cardiac rhythm specialist, in the LIJ cafeteria. In the manner of most doctors in his specialty, Tom was calm, detached, and thoughtful, and we had become friendly. I was still fuming over Davenport's and Holman's incompetence. If only they had examined my father properly, a $20,000 diagnostic workup and a great deal of worry could have easily been avoided.

Of course, I should hardly have been surprised. At one time, keen observation and the judicious laying on of hands were virtually the only diagnostic tools a doctor had. Today they seem almost obsolete. Technology like MRI scans and nuclear imaging rules the day, permitting diagnosis at a distance. Many doctors don't even carry a stethoscope anymore.

Physicians' exam skills, as a result, have no doubt atrophied. In a study I'd read about at Duke University Medical Center, a leading teaching hospital, residents in internal medicine were asked to listen to three common heart murmurs programmed into a mannequin. Roughly half could not identify two of the murmurs despite testing in a quiet room with ample time—hardly normal conditions. About two-thirds missed the third murmur. (Retesting did not improve performance.) And in another study at thirty-one internal medicine and family practice residency programs on the East Coast, over five hundred residents and medical students were tested on twelve heart sounds taped from patients. On average, the residents got only 20 percent right, not much better than the students. Hard to imagine such abysmal performances when physicians had only a stethoscope and an electrocardiograph machine to examine the heart.

The impetus behind these lapses, I'd come to believe, is that doctors today are uncomfortable with uncertainty. Everyone wants a number, a lab test, a simple objective measurement to make a diagnosis. If a physical exam can diagnose a pinched spinal nerve with only 90 percent probability, then there is an almost irresistible urge to get a thousand-dollar MRI to close the gap. Fear of lawsuits is partly to blame, but the stronger fear is that of subjective observation. Doctors are uneasy making educated guesses based on what they see and hear. If postmodernism teaches that there are many truths, or perhaps no truth, postmodern medicine teaches the opposite: that an objective truth is sure to explain a patient's symptoms if only we look for it with the right tools.

Under a flashing art deco coffee cup, I told Tom a story that an old-timer cardiologist at NYU had once told me. A group of residents had presented to him a case of atrial fibrillation, an abnormal heart rhythm, replete with results of echocardiograms, angiograms, and stress tests. He went to see the patient and immediately noticed that the whites of her eyes had black discoloration, a sign of a potentially serious metabolic derangement. No doctor had commented on it during the presentation. "I did a . . . hello!" the cardiologist recalled. "How could they have missed it? All through the chart was written 'pupils equally round and reactive to light.' It was obvious no one had examined her. I subscribe to the Yogi Berra School of physical diagnosis. You can learn a lot by looking."

Tom smiled, slowly chewing his scrambled eggs. "I majored in music in college," he said. "Knowing how to separate sounds and time them correctly has helped me immensely in listening to the heart. It'd be a shame if we lost those diagnostic skills. When you think of all the useless things we learn in medical school, physical diagnosis probably isn't one of them."

Then he added: "By the time patients get to me, they have already seen their internist and cardiologist. They have had their echos and caths. Still, I feel an obligation to examine them. When I listen to their hearts, I make sure to put my hand on their shoulder to convey a sense of warmth. I think it is enormously important to touch patients before I cut into them."

———

I made my own mistakes that first year as an attending physician. There was so much to keep track of, it was hard to know where to start—or stop. I had to master billing codes, make a template for consultation letters, learn which procedures got reimbursed (six-minute walk, sleep apnea screening, external counterpulsation), and tap into community resources (support groups, visiting nurse service, home hospice). A doctor I'd met at a conference for graduating cardiology fellows told me that since I likely wasn't going to generate even a fraction of the revenue of procedure-based cardiologists in my department, I should at least keep track of downstream earnings on catheterizations and pacemakers I ordered for my patients, so I came up with a scheme to do that, too. Then there was the actual work of patient care. Should I document every abnormality in that stack of EKGs? Should I try to master the specifics of this particular case or cede turf to the residents? As an attending you had to know how to toggle back and forth between a bird's-eye view and the details. Delegation was the key. Sometimes it helped to ask, What would I do if this were my father? It was always interesting to note which insights—such as *Do we really need another test to make this diagnosis?*—would pop into your head when you asked yourself that basic question.

I had manifold responsibilities at the hospital. As the director of the heart failure program I was accountable for the overall care the hospital provided to patients with this disease. Though it is often difficult to treat, heart failure has a characteristic physiology. In most cases it begins with an acute decrease in the heart's pumping function. The weakened heart is unable to propel blood out of the lungs, resulting in plasma leakage into the air spaces, which causes decreased oxygen tension and shortness of breath. At the same time, blood pressure drops, as the heart is unable to maintain a normal cardiac output, resulting in fatigue and damage to vital organs, especially the kidneys. Heart failure treatments, such as diuretics for removing excess salt and bodily fluid, attempt to counteract, however inadequately, these effects.

More than half a million Americans develop congestive heart failure every year. It is the number one reason patients over sixty-five years of age are hospitalized. The problem is growing: the number of hospital admissions for heart failure has more than doubled in the past two decades to more than one million. Not long ago these patients might have died of their disease, but now, as medicine has advanced, they are able to live with it. (Ironically, as medicine becomes more successful at treating sickness, the set of people who are ill is growing.) The total cost of treating the disease is more than $40 billion per year, and the majority of patients still die within five years of diagnosis.

To improve inpatient heart failure management, I wrote up a standardized physicians' order set for use in the emergency room. I put together a "care map," a formalized treatment algorithm, for nurses. I met frequently with clinical staff, trying to discover ways to improve treatment. A big problem was a lack of health literacy—patients not knowing that they needed to eliminate salt from their diets or take their medications regularly, for example—which was due in no small part to inadequate teaching on the part of their care providers. A typical complaint from patients was that their doctors had told them they had weak hearts but never told them why. "I spent two weeks in the hospital, but no one ever talked to me about it," one patient told me. "They never said, 'This is what is happening. This is what you can expect.' In fact, no one ever talked to me about it until now."

At a clinical team meeting one morning, a Haitian nurse asked me rhetorically: "So do the private doctors go into the room and explain to the patients what they have? Well, I'll tell you, they don't. It is my contention that they don't get the proper education, and that's why their care suffers."

"It's not all the doctors' fault," another nurse countered. "Sometimes I blame the patient. You go in there and they got a million questions, but when the doctor goes in there, they say everything's fine. They don't want to ask the doctor anything."

"And why is that?" I asked.

"Because they have a relationship with me," the nurse replied. "They don't have a relationship with the doctor, especially if he's just seeing them in the hospital. Doctors come and go. They don't really talk." The Haitian nurse nodded vigorously in agreement.

Those first few months at LIJ, a large number of my inpatient consults came from Rajiv because he would accept horribly sick patients from other hospitals (his motto was "Just say yes"), then dump them onto the heart failure service. Apart from taking the initial call and occasionally catheterizing the patients he accepted, he rarely took care of them, leaving that responsibility to clinical cardiologists like me. The fellows groused. They had to do most of the work managing these train wrecks.

Though I was an employee of the hospital, my salary, as with all physicians at LIJ, was linked to how much revenue I generated (though not nearly as directly as if I'd been working for myself in private practice).

"On January first, everyone talks about research and teaching," Rajiv warned me when I started. "But on December thirty-first, they only want to know how much money you've brought in." The revenue was measured in terms of "relative value unit" collections. RVUs define the values insurers place on medical services. For the past twenty years a committee (called the Relative Value Scale Update Committee, or RUC) comprised of twenty-nine physician representatives from the major medical societies has proposed specific RVU amounts for seven thousand medical services. (Though the recommendations are only suggestions, history shows that they have almost always been accepted by Centers for Medicare & Medicaid Services [CMS], the agency that administers Medicare and Medicaid, and not long thereafter by private insurers.) The RVUs are multiplied by a conversion factor (currently about $35 per RVU) to come up with the dollar amount physicians receive as payment for their work (with some adjustments made for geographical cost differences). For example, a moderately complex outpatient visit (coded 99213) is valued at 2.0 RVUs by Medicare and reimbursed about $70. Therefore, a general internist who sees fifteen moderately complex patients six days a week for forty-eight weeks out of the year, after subtracting office overhead (rent, staff salaries, malpractice insurance, and other expenses) of 50 percent of total revenue (a reasonable average for most physicians), will earn about $150,000 a year before taxes. (The first ten patients each day just cover practice costs.) Primary care physicians have often complained that representation on the RUC is tilted toward specialists, who have weighted reimbursement rates away from evaluation and management services (basically office and hospital visits) and toward procedures. Others have criticized CMS for allowing its payment rates to be determined by the very group that receives those payments.

Whatever the economics, I quickly learned that it was important to see as many patients as possible. The talk around the hospital those first few months was "Rajiv's brother has opened shop; let's give him some business." On the wards, doctors—even cardiothoracic surgeons who might have dismissed me a few months prior, when I was still a cardiology fellow—frequently stopped me to say hello. ("So you're the famous Dr. Jauhar! I've been seeing your name on charts all over the hospital." "No, that's my brother, Rajiv.") One afternoon I met a Korean internist with a stained shirt and bad breath who talked to me about the merits of being a hospital employee. "Basically, you're trading income for security," he explained. Hospital employment offered a guaranteed salary and a better work-life balance. Private practice—where doctors are independent contractors endeavoring for themselves—typically required longer hours but was rewarded with higher earnings.

"Do you ever think about private practice?" I asked.

He laughed. "Not anymore. My wife tells me all the time, 'You don't know how to be social, drum up business.' It's easier when you start off private, but once you start working for a hospital, it is hard to develop."

"So you're here for the long haul?"

"Yes, I am institutionalized," he replied with a grin. "It's like that movie *The Shawshank Redemption*. He was in prison for so long he didn't know what to do when he got out."

I mentioned what Rajiv had told me were the three attributes of a successful private practitioner: accessibility, availability, and affability.

"I heard there was another one," he said coldly. "Average."

The subject of private practice was a frequent topic of discussion in the doctors' lounge, where private practitioners and hospital employees frequently sat to discuss cases or business over a cup of coffee. Dr. Mukherjee, a pulmonologist, had quit his hospital job for private practice about two years prior. "Initially you're excited because it's something new," I heard him tell another doctor, a kidney specialist, "but time passes, and then slowly you start to think, What nonsense am I doing?"

The kidney doctor laughed. "I was told that a more profitable career than being a physician is pole dancing," she said. "So I've been trying to get slim going up and down the stairs."

In November, with Sonia (who had deferred taking a job so she could take care of our newborn) and Mohan back in our apartment and comfortably in their daily routine—bath, nap, park, nap, etc.—I started to spend more time at work. I was getting busier at the hospital. My department finally hired a nurse practitioner for me, John Meister, a congenial man who had worked as a CCU nurse for over twenty years. Nurse practitioners have advanced nursing degrees and licenses that allow them to work at least partly independently of physicians (they can write drug prescriptions, for example). John had earned his degree about two years before we met. He was a stocky fellow of German descent beloved by his colleagues, inspiring greetings in the corridors from everyone from hospital executives to senior physicians to the custodial staff. He had earned all manner of nursing awards, including twice being named nurse of the year at LIJ. He told me that at the cardiologist's office where he'd previously worked part-time, patients with virtually any complaint would get a standard panel of expensive cardiac tests: echocardiogram, Holter monitor, nuclear stress test. "And that's even if you're young and have only, say, one risk factor for heart disease," he said. Of course, the tests have utility in the proper clinical situation, but in young people they are often unnecessary. Disillusioned by the mercenary nature of private practice, he'd decided to quit and work as a salaried employee at the hospital full-time.

Together John and I saw inpatients every day and outpatients three times a week. John saw them first, getting their histories and examining them; then we saw them together. (The more redundancy in our interactions, I figured, the less chance that something would get missed.) Ours were complicated patients who required a lot of attention, and it came as no surprise that private physicians, pressed for time, were referring them to us.

Harold Peters was one such gentleman, an eighty-seven-year-old who came to my office every couple of months, faithfully accompanied by his daughter. He had severely elevated blood pressure in his lungs, a result of congestive heart failure, causing him to feel terribly fatigued and short of breath. When I told him I could put him on an expensive new drug to treat the disease, he immediately dismissed the idea. "What's the point, Doc?" he said. "What's the point of a drug that costs the government thirty-eight hundred dollars a month? Isn't it selfish?"

"What about the patient?" his daughter demanded.

"Yeah, well, I guess some people want to stay alive as long as possible. Not me. What's the point of living if I can't walk? I walk just a few feet and . . . I'm gone."

"Wait, are you saying that you'd rather be dead than weak?" his daughter said.

"That's exactly what I'm saying."

"Well, we are not having this conversation anymore," she said, waving her hand. "I am not ready to be an orphan."

"See, Doc, that's what I mean. It's selfish."

He told me he was spending most of his days alone in the house he had lived in for forty-eight years.

"In all that time you didn't make any friends?" I asked gently.

"Sure I did, but . . ." His voice trailed off.

His daughter quickly filled in: "They're all dead."

He nodded dolefully. "Yes, most of my friends are dead."

"But not everyone, Daddy."

"Who's still alive?"

"Mr. Barney."

"Oh, I guess that's true. Barney's still alive."

"Can't you spend time with him?" I asked.

"Invite him over to play cards," John, the nurse practitioner, suggested.

He shook his head. "No, we are not going to play cards."

"Why not?" I asked.

"Well, let's just say that Daddy's more mentally agile than Mr. Barney."

"So let him win!" John cried.

Patients came to us with a range of complaints, and not always concerning their physical hearts. Ella Gerson, whose heart was functioning at less than 30 percent of normal, told me this about her husband: "He drinks, Doctor, every afternoon, and if he doesn't have it, he gets nasty. Seven bottles at our neighborhood bar. He used to walk there, but since his stomach cancer was cut out—only a little is left—now he takes the bus. After the operation he stopped for about a month because he couldn't taste the beer, but when he got his taste back, he started drinking again." She sighed. "After so many years, I have nothing left. I asked Dr. Briggs, my primary, 'Send me to rehab.' He asked why. I said, 'To get away from my husband.'" Then she gave a sad chuckle.

I had my share of frustrations in the office. A frequent one was appeals to insurance companies to authorize office procedures, like echocardiograms. Some insurers refused to pay for certain procedures unless you called them up front. It was part of the "utilization review" introduced by managed care in the 1980s. A typical phone exchange would go something like this:

"Hi, this is Dr. Jauhar calling again for preauthorization."

"Yes, Dr. Jauhar, hold on."

A couple of minutes would pass. "None of the medical directors are available, Dr. Jauhar. Let me try to get a nurse for you."

"Well, is a nurse going to be able to approve this test?"

"I don't know if she's going to be able to approve it, Doctor. You'll have to discuss it with her . . . [blah blah blah]."

"So what are you going to do now?"

"I'm going to get someone. Hold on, Doctor."

And then, inevitably: "At the tone, please record your message. When you have finished recording, hang up or press pound for more options." Beep.

I enjoyed working with John and the fellows who rotated onto my service each month. We took care of very sick patients that most doctors at the hospital felt uncomfortable treating. We used novel drugs that few cardiologists had experience with. We brought our patients to an advanced level of care that hadn't existed before I arrived. And so we quickly succeeded in carving out a niche for ourselves.

Esther McAllister was typical of our inpatients. About sixty years old, she was admitted to the hospital with fluid overload from not taking her medications and eating too much salt. Her legs were purplish and her abdominal wall was leathery hard, both consequences of severe heart failure. She was morbidly obese, weighing 320 pounds. All the teeth of her lower jaw were missing save one, which jutted out like a fang.

"I don't know why they don't bring you the bedpan when you need it," she groused one afternoon, chewing gum like cud. Her Coke bottle spectacles lent her a schoolmarmish air. "Seems they'd rather clean up after me than give me the pan."

I dispatched a resident to fetch a nurse's aide.

"Last time I went in the bed, the man came in and said, 'Do you do that on yourself all the time?'" She shifted uncomfortably. "They'd better hurry or there's going to be another accident."

I sat down in the chair next to her bed and leafed through her chart. John and Simon, our fellow for the month, remained standing, waiting for me to initiate the conversation. She had been in the hospital for over a week. "Feels like three years," she said. "During the day, it's hot as Hades. At night you can chip off the icicles." Relieved of excess water weight, she was forty pounds lighter than she'd been on admission, breathing much better but still feeling weak with even a tiny bit of exertion.

"Have you been getting out of bed at all?" I asked her, turning a page.

"Not recently."

"Not even to the bathroom?"

She shook her head.

"Where do you go?"

"Unfortunately, in the diaper."

At home she'd been able to do most activities of daily living—bathing, dressing, preparing meals—though she'd been housebound. "I didn't want to go out," she explained. "I was feeling very down."

"Well, that will hopefully change now that it's getting warmer," I said. "It's been a rough winter. I've been a little depressed myself," I added frivolously.

She perked up. "Who hugs you, Doctor?"

I laughed. "No one." The sheer arduousness of taking care of a newborn had sapped the romantic energy at home.

"Don't look at me," John quickly interjected.

"I'll give you a hug," she said.

Embarrassed, I shook my head. "No, that's all right."

"No, it's not all right. Come here. Give me a hug."

She struggled to sit up, swaying from side to side to pull up her three hundred or so pounds. Then she grabbed hold of me. "If you get fifteen hugs a day, all your problems will be solved."

"I wish it were that easy," I said as she squeezed the air out of me.

"No, I'm serious," she said. "A hug does something to your inside." (No question about that, I thought, feeling my spleen being crushed.)

After breaking from her clench, I had her sit up so I could listen to her chest. Her thick gray chin hairs tickled the back of my hand. She smelled of cheap perfume, but the odor was inoffensive, even slightly pleasant. While I was examining her, she glanced at Simon, the cardiology fellow, standing quietly behind me.

"What do you want to be when you grow up?" she asked him.

"I'm training to be a heart doctor," he replied stiffly. "I have a couple more years."

"I wanted to be a photographer's model," she said. We all laughed, except Simon. "Do you like old movies?" she asked him.

"Sometimes," he replied, rocking nervously on his feet.

"Well, I love those old Betty Grable movies. And Marilyn Monroe, too. Did you know me and Elizabeth are only three months apart?"

"Elizabeth?" Simon said.

"Yes, Elizabeth Taylor. But we're different. I only had one husband." Simon stared at her impassively. "He was a good man," she went on. "He said, 'I'm the husband. I don't want you to work.'"

"What did you do?" I asked.

"I didn't work! What was I going to do, argue? Someone tells you, 'I'll support you,' what would you do?"

An orderly arrived with a bedpan. I told Ms. McAllister that we would come back to see her the next day.

"Okay," she said, turning onto her side so the receptacle could be placed under her bottom. She looked straight at Simon. "Smile, sweetie. It only gets worse when you get older."

———

Those first few months at LIJ, I frequently assumed attending duties in the cardiac care unit. Most of my cases were straightforward, but a few required a subtle touch. Dick Perkins, a middle-aged construction executive, was admitted to the CCU one Saturday night after a prolonged bout of chest pain. Blood tests showed he had suffered a moderate heart attack, in which blood flow to the heart muscle is cut off by a coronary blockage. But when he was told he needed a coronary angiogram, he balked. "He doesn't want any invasive procedures," a bedraggled nurse explained when I arrived for rounds on Sunday morning.

I had encountered such resistance many times. "I'll talk to him," I said. Patients are often anxious about cardiac catheterization, and a discussion of the risks and benefits usually allays their fears. But the nurse said Mr. Perkins had been ranting and uncooperative with blood draws and blood pressure checks. A psychiatrist, asked to assess decision-making ability, had deemed him incapacitated—he seemed to have paranoid delusions about his medical condition—and suggested forcibly treating him, if necessary.

I walked into his room, hoping to avoid a showdown. He was standing with his back to me, talking on a cell phone. When he heard me, he hung up and turned around; he was an overweight man with a sallow, jowly face and a potbelly, wearing Dockers and a blue oxford cloth shirt. I extended my hand. "Hi, I'm Dr. Jauhar," I said. "I'm the cardiologist on call for the weekend."

He eyed me suspiciously but reluctantly shook my hand. I asked him to sit down, but he remained standing, arms folded, with a fixed and fervent look.

"You've had a heart attack," I started off.

"So you say," he shot back.

"Well, this is something I can say with confidence," I replied, trying to project authority. "I'm told you're a building expert. I know next to nothing about buildings, so anything you tell me I am likely to believe. Similarly, I think you should trust me if I tell you that you've had a heart attack. After all, I know how to identify heart attacks. It's what I do."

I asked someone to pass me a printout of his test results. After I showed him the abnormal cardiac enzyme levels, he sneered and said: "Fine. So you think I had a heart attack." Clearly, he still did not believe me.

"The best treatment for a heart attack is angioplasty," I said.

"I don't want it," he said, his voice rising. "I told them I don't want a stent."

"No one can force you to have it," I said calmly. Angioplasty, in which tiny balloons and stents are used to relieve coronary blockages, wouldn't work without his cooperation, and I wasn't about to call in security guards to frog-march him to the catheterization lab. "But I think you should reconsider."

He glared at me and said he did not want to discuss the matter further.

"Okay," I said. "We'll watch you for another twenty-four hours. If your condition remains stable, we'll send you home."

"No, I'm leaving now." He moved to gather his things.

I watched him for a few moments. "You can't leave," I finally said.

"Who says?"

I wasn't sure how to respond. "The psychiatrist," I said tentatively.

"Which psychiatrist?" he snarled. "The little faggot with the pony-tail? The little frilly guy?"

I immediately walked out to the nurses' station and phoned Mr. Perkins's son. He explained that his father had always been "strong-willed" and "done things just the way he wanted." The behavior I was describing wasn't so different from his norm.

Now I felt even more conflicted. On the one hand, my patient clearly did not meet the standards for decision-making capacity. He did not understand his medical condition or its treatment options and the risks and benefits. If I let him sign out against medical advice and something happened to him (sudden death, another myocardial infarction), I would be liable. On the other hand, his intransigence was apparently just a part of who he was. As a doctor, I want to see my patients weigh risks and benefits in a careful, reasoned manner, use logic, have a clear sense of self, etc. In other words, I want them to think like me. But Perkins's mind operated differently from mine, and not because he was sick. Shouldn't I just allow him to be himself rather than insist on what I wanted him to be?

The situation resembled a famous medical ethics case I'd read about. In 1978, Mary Northern, a seventy-two-year-old woman in Tennessee, developed gangrene in both feet, requiring amputation. When she refused to have the surgery, doctors at Nashville General Hospital determined that she did not have decision-making capacity and filed a lawsuit for permission to amputate her legs. "Ms. Northern does not understand the severity or consequences of her disease process," they wrote to the Department of Human Services in Nashville. "[She] does not appear to understand that failure to amputate the feet at this time would probably result in her death."

A psychiatrist concurred, stating that Ms. Northern was generally sane but was psychotic with respect to ideas concerning her gangrenous feet. "She tends to believe that her feet are black because of soot or dirt," he wrote. "She does not believe her physicians about the serious infection."

Two judges from the Tennessee Supreme Court went to see Ms. Northern in the hospital. "They tell us that your feet are shriveling up like a dead person's feet," one of the judges told her.

"No, no," she replied, insisting she could get up and "walk all the way down to the shopping places."

The judge asked: "If the time comes that you have to choose between losing your feet and dying, would you rather just go ahead and die than lose your feet?"

She replied: "It's possible. It's possible only if I—just forget it. I—you are making me sick talking."

Before he left, the judge asked her, "Did you ever read the Sermon on the Mount?"

"Yes," Ms. Northern replied.

"You remember one thing the Good Lord said?"

"What?"

"If thy eye offend thee—"

"Oh, yes, take the eye out."

"—cast it out. If thy hand offend you, cut it off. Now, if and when your feet begin to offend you, maybe, maybe, you will remember that little verse."

The court decided that Ms. Northern was incompetent to make a rational decision and should have her feet amputated against her wishes. "On the subjects of death and amputation of her feet, her comprehension is blocked, blinded, or dimmed to the extent that she is incapable of recognizing facts which would be obvious to a person of normal perception," the opinion read. "If [she] would assume and exercise her rightful control over her own destiny by stating that she prefers death to the loss of her feet, her wish would be respected . . . But because of her inability or unwillingness to recognize the actual condition of her feet, she is incompetent to make a rational decision." However, because of complications, the surgery was never performed. Several months later she died as a result of a clot from her gangrenous leg that migrated to a vital organ.

That afternoon I discussed the Perkins case with a member of the hospital ethics committee. "If you say he has decision-making capacity, then you have to say that he has the right of self-determination, even if you don't agree with him," he told me. "If he lacks decision-making capacity, you first go to a surrogate. If the surrogate is unwilling to act in the patient's best interest, then courts have said that you have to do what's in your power to prevent the patient from hurting himself. So it all depends on whether you think he has decision-making capacity or not."

I believed Mr. Perkins lacked capacity because he was unable to acknowledge that he had a serious disease or to understand the risks, benefits, and alternatives of treatment. However, there was no need for drastic measures. When I threatened to call security to keep him from leaving, he backed down. Though still refusing nursing checks and cardiac monitoring, he remained in his room overnight.

When I went to see him the following morning, his demeanor had changed. He was making laps around the unit with an orderly, still refusing telemetry monitoring, blood draws, vital sign checks, and medications, but now he seemed quite pleasant and reasonable. He told me he understood that he had a heart problem but that he wanted to go home and follow up with a cardiologist as an outpatient.

It appeared to me that he had recovered decision-making capacity, and after seeing him, the psychiatrist agreed. Though still at risk, my patient had every right to sign out against medical advice. That is exactly what he did later that day.

———

I learned to make hard decisions those first few months as an attending, but the learning curve was steep. The pressure could be overwhelming at times because mistakes often had huge consequences, and fear of malpractice—and the resulting lawsuit—were lurking just under the surface of most of my and my colleagues' dealings with patients. One morning I got a call from the emergency room. A young man—an intern, in fact, who had been on rounds on the wards—had been admitted with chest pains. Could I come to evaluate him?

The ER that morning was the usual mess of drunks, druggies, and demented old ladies pretending to read *The New Yorker*. There were the usual pressured announcements overhead ("Linda, stat to the trauma bay . . . Linda"). Stretchers were arranged like latticework in the corridors, and the air was suffused with stale body odor. Searching for my patient, I ran into Joe Ricci, a jovial cardiologist who practiced in Howard Beach. Ricci was always impeccably dressed and, unlike most private practice doctors, never looked as if he was in a hurry. "How are things?" he said pleasantly. "Getting used to the place?"

I said I was. In fact, I was quite enjoying my work and was finally starting to feel confident. Ricci brought up a mutual patient. "Sarah Brenner is doing very well," he said. "I guess those drugs you're pushing really do something." I laughed. "By the way," he said conspiratorially, "did you see the article in the *Times* about how doctors should work on Sundays? Ridiculous, isn't it? They think we're selling shoes."

When I found the intern, Zahid Talwar, he was sitting on the side of a gurney, legs dangling, looking bored. He was about thirty years old, a Pakistani man with a long face and a white coat who straightened up respectfully when I arrived. I introduced myself and asked him about the chest pain. It had started after dinner the night before and had lasted about ten minutes. He had slept comfortably, but the pain recurred while he was walking to the bus stop that morning, persisting for almost an hour. It was a dense pressure in the center of his chest. To be on the safe side, he had decided to leave rounds and come to the ER.

His blood tests were normal, as was his first electrocardiogram. He had none of the traditional risk factors for heart disease, such as diabetes, hypertension, or a regular smoking habit. I suspected he was suffering from acute pericarditis, a usually benign inflammation of the membrane around the heart often treated with over-the-counter anti-inflammatory drugs. Characteristic of pericarditis, the pain worsened when he took a deep breath. I told him that if blood tests in six hours were normal, we would send him home. I joked there were easier ways to get out of internship duty.

Later that morning I got a call from an ER physician informing me that my patient's pain had resolved completely after he had taken ibuprofen, further confirming the diagnosis of pericarditis. For a moment I considered sending him home right then, but I decided to wait until the next set of blood tests was complete.

Just before leaving the hospital that evening, I ran into a physician's assistant. He told me that Zahid's subsequent blood tests showed evidence of minor cardiac muscle damage. This took me by surprise. Pericarditis usually does not result in abnormal cardiac enzyme levels. I quickly explained that the problem was probably myopericarditis, in which inflammation of the surrounding membrane can partially involve the heart muscle. He asked me if the young doctor should have a cardiac catheterization to rule out coronary blockages. It was late; I told him that any workup could wait until morning. I assured him that a thirty-year-old with no risk factors did not have coronary artery disease. I instructed him to draw more enzymes and to order an echocardiogram and call me at home if there were problems.

Zahid had chest pains through the night. Doctors who were called to see him attributed them to myopericarditis, the diagnosis I had written in the chart. At 2:00 a.m. he asked for more ibuprofen. "I told them, if it's pericarditis, give me more medication," he told me later. "Means, do whatever it takes to make the pain go away."

When I saw him in the morning, the pain had subsided. However, further blood tests showed evidence of continuing heart muscle injury, and an EKG showed nonspecific abnormalities. Though I still doubted that he had coronary disease, I sent him to the cardiac catheterization lab for an angiogram.

I received a call from Rajiv about an hour later, asking me to come over to the lab. When I arrived, the angiogram was playing on a computer screen. It showed a complete blockage of the left anterior descending artery, the so-called widow-maker lesion. The artery looked like a lobster tail, unnaturally terminating after several centimeters. X-rays showed severe dysfunction of the entire anterior portion of the left ventricle. My patient had been having a full-blown heart attack, in which blood flow to the front part of his heart had entirely ceased, damaging the muscle, for more than twenty-four hours.

Nurses were spinning in swivel chairs, impatiently waiting for Rajiv to start the stent procedure. I sat down on a stool, feeling weak. Even the beeping in the control room sounded like an admonition. Rajiv was wearing a lead apron, standing over my patient, who was lying on a narrow operating table behind X-ray-opaque glass. Rajiv stared at me for a few seconds, as if trying to gauge my reaction. "Arm the dye injector, please," he called out to a nurse.

"Done," she replied.

"Give me ten cc's of dye for twenty seconds."

"Coming up."

"Can I have a three-millimeter stent?"

"You got it."

And then, before I knew it, he had inflated a balloon and deployed the stent, restoring blood flow down the coronary artery. "All right, I'm done," he announced.

Afterward, heat rose to my face as colleagues wandered in to inquire about what was going on. I said little, other than that my patient's symptoms had mimicked pericarditis. But what I was thinking was, You bastard, how could you have missed it? I was well aware of the disturbing prevalence of heart disease in South Asians, whose risk is up to four times that of other ethnic groups. I knew that heart attacks in this population frequently occurred in men under forty years of age, who often don't exhibit classic coronary risk factors. I knew all this, but somehow my mind had suffered a block. So much for the expertise I had claimed with Mr. Perkins.

"Don't beat yourself up," a colleague said sympathetically. "Every doctor I know would have done the same thing." Another told me that it was his policy to "cath" almost anyone who came to the ER complaining of chest pains. In his opinion, the risks posed by routine coronary angiograms were much less than that of a missed heart attack.

Rajiv came out of the procedure room and took me aside. "It could have happened to anybody," he said quietly, "but now don't try to justify it."

I started to blame the on-call fellow, who'd gotten information during the night to diagnose the myocardial infarction, but Rajiv stopped me. "It's not his ass on the line," he said. "That's the difference now."

"I'm not sure I did anything wrong," I replied weakly. "Even Andrew said anyone could have—"

"Andrew thinks you fucked up, all right," Rajiv snapped. "He's just being nice. Look, it happened. Just admit you fucked up and don't talk about it."

I looked through the glass at my patient, being wheeled out of the lab.

"People love it when shit happens to somebody," Rajiv explained. "This morning I had a stent complication. The patient was coding on the table. I was thinking, Fuck, the patient is going to die, I'm going to feel bad, I'll have to talk to the family, lawsuit, paperwork, et cetera, et cetera, but the fellows loved it. It's like NASCAR races: they go round and round in a fucking circle, big deal. But when there's an accident, everyone gets excited."

What now? I knew I had to explain myself, but how much should I say? I had made errors before, but never one this big—and only a short while on the job, too. Should I just tell my patient the facts? Should I apologize?

Most doctors are afraid to take responsibility for medical errors. We are acutely aware of the potential hazards—legal and professional—of taking ownership of a mistake. In surveys most doctors say medical errors should be reported, but a large number don't report their own, especially minor ones that do not cause disability or death. "Apologies are a means of being polite if you are seven years old," a doctor wrote on Sermo, the physician online community. "But when you are in medical practice, it has little role in patient care. An apology says, when the smoke clears, 'I'm too inexperienced to be doing what I did.' And, whether we like it or not, that is precisely what patients, their attorneys, and juries hear."

Another doctor wrote: "The whole 'apologize and hope it goes away' thing is such a phony myth perpetuated by ethics types who don't have to worry about career ruin in the lawyer gang-bang that is U.S. health care." And another wrote: "It's like confessing an extramarital affair to your spouse. What do you expect to accomplish?"

However, studies have shown that physicians' apologies do not necessarily increase malpractice lawsuits. In fact, they might protect against litigation. In surveys patients say they desire acknowledgment of even minor errors. For both moderate and severe mistakes, patients are significantly more likely to sue if a physician does not disclose the error, a fact most doctors are unaware of.

There has been a trend toward such apologies. Twenty-nine states have enacted legislation encouraging them, some even making physicians' expressions of remorse inadmissible in court. It wasn't always this way. Hospital legal departments routinely used to advise doctors never to admit responsibility for errors. During my internship orientation, a lawyer for the hospital said that at some point in our careers every one of us would likely be sued, and that we could even be sued during residency. She offered some advice: document your decision-making; document when a patient refuses treatment; never admit wrongdoing; never talk to an opposing attorney; and finally, be nice to your patients. Doctors who were nice to their patients were rarely sued, even in cases of egregious malpractice.

I couldn't bring myself to talk to my patient in the cath lab, while everyone was watching, so I decided to wait until he got to the recovery room, where it was more private. I found him there lying on a stretcher. The pain in his chest was gone, he happily informed me. However, the groin where the catheter had been inserted now hurt. "They substituted one pain for another," he said, laughing.

I grasped the side rails of the gurney. "I thought you had pericarditis," I said carefully. I paused. "I was obviously wrong. I'm sorry."

He seemed embarrassed. "No, no, please, the past is finished," he replied. "I am more interested in the future." He asked me why this had happened; his cholesterol level was normal. I explained that there were many factors besides cholesterol—some we didn't even know about—

that were at play. He inquired about his prognosis. I told him that I thought it was good, though because of the significant damage that had occurred to his heart—damage made worse, no doubt (though I didn't tell him this), because of my misdiagnosis—he would have to be on medications for the rest of his life. He nodded, looking disappointed.

A few days later, just before he was to be discharged, I stopped by his room. I asked him with whom he was going to follow up. He told me that he had been given the name of another cardiologist but that he had decided to go with me. "You have been terrific," he said. "Thank you for everything."

I nodded silently, feeling empty. "You are much too generous," I said.

FOUR

Good Intentions

In nothing do men more nearly approach the gods than in giving
health to men.
           —Cicero

The arguments started soon after Mohan was born, and though they
were ostensibly about my job and our lack of disposable income, and not
so much about the added responsibilities of a new baby, they were really
about our future, what sort of lives we wanted to lead, and so, in fact,
they really were about Mohan after all.

"I don't think it's asking a lot for you to think about our future," Sonia said one evening after I had put Mohan to bed. "Your hours are
similar to Rajiv's, and yet we are struggling financially. That is why I am
bringing up private practice."

I tried to explain that Rajiv, whose salary was at least double mine,
performed invasive procedures, lucratively reimbursed in our current
system, but Sonia didn't want to hear about how the American medical
payment model should change.

"You think this is about jewelry or a four-car garage? Have I asked for
those things?"

She had not, but we couldn't afford them anyway. The glum reality
was that we were cash poor. After we paid rent and student loans, there
was very little left over. We had enough money to entertain desires—a
car for Sonia to drive to New Jersey to visit her parents, for example—
but not nearly enough to realize them.

"I told you I don't want to do private practice," I said firmly. "It has
nothing to do with you or how I feel about—"

"But it does, because we are a family. And we are crammed into a tiny one-bedroom apartment!"

A force was bearing down on me, pinning me to the headboard of the bed. I wanted to holler, but I didn't have the energy to deal with the inevitably ugly aftermath. "I can't do it," I said, though with less conviction than before.

"Of course you can! You considered it during your fellowship. Why don't you talk to my father? He could guide us—"

"I don't want to do private practice!" I shouted. "Those guys are a bunch of crooks. I see it every day in the hospital."

Sonia's father, a pulmonologist, had made his money in the era after Medicare was introduced. Like most doctors of that generation, he had learned to play the fee-for-service game, amassing a huge personal fortune—millions—the kind of money that wasn't available anymore, no matter how hard you worked. He had told me I was living in a fool's paradise as a salaried physician, where there was little financial incentive to see more patients or order tests. "If you want to get ghee out of a jar, you cannot do it with a straight finger," he'd said, recounting an old Punjabi proverb. "It has to be bent." But I didn't want to do private practice. I didn't want to give up my job and the academic life, where I could practice the way I wanted, mostly free from the demands of the marketplace; where there was no pressure to overtreat patients; and where I could take pride in teaching the next generation of doctors. Ironically, it's the people who have money who seem to feel most strongly that you need money to be happy.

"I'm just asking for a plan for a better financial future," Sonia pressed on. "I know I need to work, but I can't do that right now with the baby. I want nice things for us: a home, safe cars, good schools. They may seem trivial to you, but they are not to me."

Of course, they weren't trivial, and in fact I felt sorry for my wife, overwhelmed, physically exhausted, and trapped in a shoebox apartment among piles of laundry with no room to move—and all of it under the shackle of financial dependence on me. But I believed that I couldn't allow myself to empathize. I was afraid that if I gave credence to her perceptions, I'd have to compromise what I felt at the time were my principles.

"I like my job," I said evenly. "I'm not saying that I want to be a hospital employee for the rest of my life or that I would even stay at LIJ, for that matter—"

"But it isn't just about you anymore; there is also us to think about. Getting hung up on your title isn't fair or wise for the future."

"Your father—"

"—is not your enemy. He just wants us to have the best life possible with the least stress."

"He doesn't understand—"

"What's to understand? Money is important."

"Money doesn't buy happiness."

"Yes, it does!"

And when things devolved to that degree, I knew it was time to stop, and so did she.

———

One morning in October 2004, about three months after I'd started my job, a sales representative of the pharmaceutical company Scios came into my office and made me an offer I found hard to refuse. She invited me to join Scios's speakers' bureau and start giving paid talks using company slides to promote the drug Natrecor. Scios was marketing Natrecor, a synthetic version of a naturally occurring hormone, for the treatment of acute heart failure. It was a drug I had come to rely on for many of my hospitalized patients, especially the sickest ones in the CCU. A few months earlier, after I'd accepted my position at LIJ but before I'd started working as an attending, a Scios rep had contacted me at NYU, where I was finishing up my cardiology fellowship, and suggested that I consider starting a Natrecor infusion clinic when I arrived at LIJ. Though there was little data recommending the use of the drug in office patients, outpatient infusion clinics for the drug were proliferating across the country because reimbursement was so profitable. The Food and Drug Administration had classified the drug as a protein-based biological agent, so Medicare was paying for its off-label administration on the same generous pay scale as chemotherapy.

I took a couple of days to think about the sales rep's speaking offer. Though I had no interest in starting an infusion clinic, especially without more data to support its use, I decided that I didn't have a problem lecturing about the drug. Though the talks were obviously for marketing purposes, I didn't think giving them would be sleazy or unethical, especially since Natrecor was a drug I prescribed and believed in. Moreover, and just as important, I needed the money. I asked my department head about it. She replied that she didn't police her faculty on such matters. So a few days later I called the rep and accepted her invitation.

This started a series of talks I gave over the next two years. At first I asked to use my own slides to maintain some semblance of objectivity, but the company wouldn't allow it. I asked if I could modify the standard company slides with some of my own interpretations, but it wouldn't allow that either. Typically, the talks took place at a fancy restaurant on Long Island or in Manhattan once or twice every couple of months. I'd get paid a thousand dollars or more for each talk. The extra money really helped. My salary as an academic cardiologist was about a third lower than if I'd been working in private practice, and since I was the sole earner for my family, the talks took some pressure off me financially. The dinners were uniformly excellent, with fine wines flowing freely. Occasionally, if I didn't feel like driving, I would even get a car service to and from the venue. The drug reps who showed up at my talks were always pretty and flirtatious. They seemed to take a genuine interest in me and my work. So I became addicted to the talks and slyly hinted at more invitations when Scios reps came detailing at my office to promote their drug.

Of course, I had mixed feelings about the whole thing. Sometimes the promised audience wouldn't materialize—doctors who were supposed to come would have to stay late in their offices—but I'd get paid anyway. I often wondered what my colleagues in the department—very few of whom had been invited to join a speakers' bureau—thought of what I was doing.

In March 2006, about a year and a half after I had started giving these talks, a paper linking Natrecor to increased mortality in acute heart failure patients was published in *The Journal of the American Medical Association*. It was a flawed study, a retrospective analysis pooling several different trials with diverse patient populations. Still, it caused a major stir. The pharmaceuticals and therapeutics committee at LIJ held an unscheduled meeting to discuss the drug, to which I was invited. At the meeting I reiterated what I believed to be true: that Natrecor was safe and effective in the right patients (those who had adequate blood pressure, no significant kidney dysfunction, etc.). I presented some slides—actually modified company slides—criticizing the paper and pointing out its many flaws. I realized that my presentation was skewed to confer maximal advantage to Scios, and I wondered whether the committee was taking me seriously or viewing me as a company pawn, which is how I was beginning to feel. Afterward the head of the committee pointedly noted that I was in Scios's speakers' bureau. Though he didn't say it explicitly, the clear implication was that my assessment was being influenced by money. In the end, the committee decided to restrict Natrecor use to me (the resident heart failure specialist) and a handful of other cardiologists. By then I'd tapered off the talks anyway, and soon afterward I quit the speakers' bureau. (A randomized, controlled trial later showed that Natrecor was safe but no more effective than existing, cheaper therapies.)

During the two years I gave these talks, I often thought of what Jacob Hirsch, a cardiologist at NYU, once told me when we were sitting in the echo reading room during my fellowship. He was eating a sandwich that had been brought in by a drug rep. "It's not the doctors at the academic centers that they should be policing," he said. "It's the docs out in the suburbs, in Long Island and New Jersey. They're the ones you have to worry about."

———

In December 2004, about six months into my first year at LIJ, John and I drove to Columbia-Presbyterian Medical Center in Manhattan to take a daylong course on artificial heart pumps and cardiac transplantation. Artificial hearts had fascinated me ever since I was a boy. I still remember watching news reports about Barney Clark, the retired dentist with end-stage heart failure who received the world's first permanent artificial heart, a refrigerator-size machine, on December 1, 1982, at the University of Utah Medical Center. I remember eagerly awaiting the latest updates on his condition while my father tsk-tsked about the poor man's fate. Though he opened his eyes and moved his limbs immediately after the operation, Clark's postoperative course was rocky. On day 3 his chest had to be reopened because of subcutaneous emphysema, a complication of surgery. On days 4 and 5 he developed progressive kidney failure. On day 6 he had generalized seizures and ended up in a coma for almost two weeks. On day 13 his prosthetic mitral valve malfunctioned and had to be replaced. Other complications followed, including respiratory failure requiring a tracheostomy tube, aspiration pneumonia, pseudomembranous colitis, and sepsis. On day 92, William DeVries, the lead surgeon, spoke with Clark in a videotaped interview. "It's been hard, hasn't it, Barney?" DeVries said. "Yes, it's been hard," Clark replied, "but the heart itself is pumping right along." It continued to pump until he finally succumbed to multiorgan failure on day 112.

Clark's Jarvik-7 was medicine's *Sputnik*; never before had a medical innovation sparked such furious debate, even a kind of national reckoning. Though the experiment was viewed as successful by some (notably Clark himself, who said he believed the operation would be "worth it" if it staved off death), most people were deeply disturbed by what they had witnessed. For some, the human heart has special spiritual and emotional meanings that made it impossible to replace with a man-made device. (Una Loy, Clark's wife of thirty-nine years, voiced this conviction when she asked, "Will he still be able to love me?") Others were troubled by the fact that Clark had never left the hospital. He survived for almost four months. But had he really lived?

Today the outlook for end-stage heart failure patients has changed considerably. The workhorse of mechanical support is the left ventricular assist device, made of plastic and titanium, which piggybacks onto the native heart and pumps blood directly out of the heart and into the aorta, which transports it to the body. LVADs (pronounced "el-vads") can help bridge patients to a heart transplant (though approximately a hundred thousand Americans could potentially benefit from heart transplantation, only two thousand donor hearts become available every year), as well as serve as a final (or "destination") therapy in those who are not transplant candidates. The devices can be implanted into a small surgical pocket in the abdomen or even in the sac around the heart, reducing the risk of bleeding and infection. The newest-generation devices can function for several years before failing. Some patients have experienced full cardiac recovery with these devices so that they can be removed, though the mechanisms remain unclear. I wanted to introduce this therapy at LIJ, and John and I had come to the right place to get trained. Columbia-Presbyterian is probably the best heart failure center on the East Coast, if not in the country.

I had spent several months at Columbia during my final year of fellowship, so I remembered well the mess of traffic and food carts that we encountered in front of the Milstein Pavilion that winter morning. Inside the marble lobby, we were met by Santo Russo, a young Italian cardiologist I had worked with. Santo was a handsome, wiry man who, despite his ill-fitting clothes and unfashionable ties, still managed to maintain a dashing air. Though he had completed his fellowship only a few years earlier, his gentle manner and good European common sense—he was pragmatic, direct, rational—made him someone I looked up to and aspired to emulate. He always had a lot to say about the hospital and American medical education. "Medical school teaches people the bad lesson that in order to succeed, you have to memorize," he'd once told me. "People go through four years of medical school, three years of residency, three years of subspecialty fellowship, and they are never taught to think. Then all of a sudden at the end of fellowship, they are told to start doing basic or clinical research. 'What do you mean, you don't know the relevant research question? We don't care that for nine years you were taught not to ask questions, to accept the prevailing wisdom. We don't care about that. We want you to start doing research!' A better way"— he'd gone on facetiously—"would be to teach medical students for six days of the week and on the seventh day make them forget everything they've learned because it will soon be outdated anyway."

Santo, John, and I stopped at a small café, where we ordered cappuccinos and chatted about my fledgling heart failure program. Then Santo took us on his rounds. In the cardiothoracic intensive care unit was a patient who had been implanted with an LVAD about a week prior, despite evidence of an overwhelming infection. "He was making almost no urine," Santo said in his slightly accented English. "Now look." The urine in his catheter bag was brown and foamy, like beer. Santo marveled at his patient's progress. "It really amazes me," he said as we stood outside the dense semicircle of machines arrayed around the bed. "We can control physiology to such minute detail that even something like sepsis, which we have been taught does not respond to our manipulations, seems to get better."

After rounds we joined up with doctors and nurse practitioners from other hospitals and attended a series of lectures. We spent the afternoon in the "cow lab," a dissection suite, where we watched a surgeon implant an LVAD into the chest of a calf. (A sign read: DON'T TAKE YOUR ORGANS TO HEAVEN . . . HEAVEN KNOWS WE NEED THEM HERE.) The calf's thorax was splayed open to reveal a pink beating heart embellished with yellow lines of fat, like a buoy in a red lake. Standing over the animal was a cardiothoracic surgeon, whose gloved fingers were moving purposefully in the chest cavity. The calf had obviously come straight from the farm because there was still mud on its hooves. A dreadlocked anesthetist was adjusting knobs on a baffle delivering intravenous medications. A technician was playing with dials on the heart-lung machine. A nurse instructed us about the various operations of the LVAD, how to change the pumping rate, how to replace the batteries, and so on. When the surgeon relaxed the aortic cross-clamp, inky droplets sprayed onto the brown and white fur. After coring out a thick piece of heart muscle about the size of a quarter, he inserted the inflow port of the LVAD into the apex of the left ventricle and stitched it in to get a blood-tight seal. Then the pump was turned on. Soon it was putting out four liters of blood per minute, enough to sustain life.

But then the calf's heart started to beat erratically and the cardiac output plummeted. Someone called for a defibrillator. The surgeon inserted the paddles into the chest and applied a 100-joule shock. The heart continued to fibrillate, so he tried 150, 200, and 300 joules, with no success. With each shock the hooves lifted off the table and the smell of grilled meat grew stronger. "Anybody bring any barbecue sauce?" someone quipped. After about ten minutes the code was stopped, and we were left with a humming LVAD inside a dead cow. The whole experience, my first with an LVAD, left me feeling a little sick.

In the men's locker room, I changed out of my bloodied scrubs. Before leaving the hospital, I went to say goodbye to Santo in the CCU. I had spent a lot of time in the CCU the previous year, and all the nurses remembered me.

At bed 10, now empty, the sad memory of James Irey came flooding back. Irey hailed from Trinidad, and though he had spent much of his adult life in the ragtag South Bronx, he retained a calm, elegant Caribbean manner. When I first met him in the emergency room at Columbia-Presbyterian, it was immediately obvious he was near the end of his life. He had congestive heart failure because of sarcoidosis, a chronic disease that infiltrates the heart and lungs with inflammatory cells. In his late fifties, bony thin, with salt-and-pepper braids, he was lying on a gurney in an almost meditative pose, as if his focusing on his labored breathing were crowding out all distractions. A combined heart-lung transplant was probably his only hope to live longer than a few months, but when I brought it up, he refused to consider it. He said he would rather die than undergo such an invasive treatment.

After reviewing the case with my colleagues, I told Irey that he needed a right heart catheterization, in which a thin, flexible tube is threaded through a vein in the groin and into the right side of the heart to measure the pressures inside the heart and lungs. Data from the catheterization would help us treat Irey medically, but just as important—though I didn't tell him this—the data would help us determine whether he was eligible for a transplant. If the pressures were too high, then for technical reasons a transplant would not be feasible. What was the harm, I thought, in getting more information? Why not just do the evaluation and deal with his objections later?

With prodding from his wife, Irey reluctantly agreed, and he underwent the procedure the following day. In the early evening I reviewed the results with Santo, my attending that month. Poring over the catheterization report, Santo pointed out a critical discrepancy in the measurements. The pressure in Irey's lungs was high, but whether the elevation was reversible or not—a crucial factor in deciding if he was a transplant candidate—was open to interpretation. To settle the issue, Santo said, the procedure would have to be repeated. Initially I demurred, wondering if it was worth doing, given Irey's opposition to a transplant, but Santo insisted we try to convince Irey, for his own sake.

We went to talk to Irey. He was in bed, wearing bright red pajamas, a stark contrast with the air of grim expectation that permeated the room. Thin plastic tubing delivering supplemental oxygen pressed tightly against his sunken cheeks, ending in tiny prongs jutting into flaring brown nostrils. His wife was with him, sitting quietly; she barely acknowledged us when we entered. Santo greeted Irey and asked him how he was feeling. Irey replied that he was still uncomfortable, especially in the right upper quadrant of the abdomen (where fluid was probably backing up in his liver because of heart failure) and that he was so exhausted he could hardly move. He inquired about the results of the catheterization. Santo matter-of-factly told him that the measurements were inconclusive and would have to be repeated.

Irey closed his eyes. "I can't go through that again," he rasped softly.

His wife started to speak, but he stopped her. "Just treat me with medicines."

"Yes, well, we are going to do that," Santo replied with his slight Italian accent. "But if you require a transplant, then we will need that information."

"No transplant," Irey said, shaking his head. He said it with even more conviction than he had the previous evening. He asked how long he could live without one.

"You are very sick," Santo said gravely. "I cannot really say, but your life span will be limited."

"How limited?" Irey said. He seemed prepared to hear even the worst prognosis.

"The most severe problem is with your lungs," Santo said. "We are not lung experts, so you really should ask the pulmonologists."

"I'm asking for your opinion. How long do I have?"

Santo shrugged. "Maybe a year," he said.

Irey didn't miss a beat. "That's fine, I'll take it. No transplant. And so I won't have to have the procedure tomorrow?"

Santo shot me a glance conveying he understood that convincing Irey would be more difficult than he had originally imagined. Leaning against a bedside table, where Irey's dinner tray was sitting untouched, he said, "Well, probably not. If you say 'no transplant,' then it puts a different light on this hospitalization."

"Then I can go home?"

"May I ask why you don't want a transplant?"

"I don't want to go through that," Irey said, waving off the idea. "I don't want anyone cutting me open."

"Your lungs are scarred," Santo began to explain. "There is a lot of fibrosis—"

"But you will still treat me?" Irey interrupted.

"But this is not what I would call treatment," Santo replied. "It is more, if you can understand what I mean, palliation." The look in Irey's eyes told me he understood. "It is like giving Tylenol for a fever. You give the Tylenol and the fever goes away, but you are not any better."

"But you will still treat me?" Irey pressed. "If I say no, you will still give me treatment to help me live as long as possible?"

"Well, yes, of course," Santo said with a trace of exasperation, as if the question were absurd. "But there is treatment at the medical level and treatment at the transplant level. There is only so much we can do without a transplant. When you crash an engine, sometimes you can fix it, but sometimes the whole thing has to be replaced. This is the situation that you are now in. If it was just your heart, we could treat it. But your lungs are the more serious problem. That you will have to discuss with the lung specialists. They will talk to you tomorrow. I hope you will have a similar conversation with them as we are having today."

"But you say one year," Irey said hopefully.

"I don't know," Santo replied quickly. "It could be less. You must ask the lung doctors. I don't want you to say, 'Dr. Russo told me I have one year to live.' Let us just say, a few months to one year."

"I understand," Irey said, settling back, looking more relaxed. "I won't tell anyone."

Mrs. Irey had a world-weary look, as if she had heard this discussion many times before. "Our understanding was that he could be put on a transplant list, and then we could decide," she said.

Santo shook his head. "It does not work that way," he said. "We need a firm commitment from the patient before we can put him on the list."

"But how can he commit when he doesn't know what it means medically?" Mrs. Irey asked. I glanced at Irey, who appeared spent and preoccupied once again with his breathing.

"That is fine, but he has to buy into the concept," Santo said. "Even then there is a low chance he will be accepted. For technical reasons we may not be able to—"

"Please forgive me for being so blunt," Mrs. Irey interrupted, "but in your opinion, would it be worth the effort? Will he be better-off?" Irey looked away, as if he had heard this line of inquiry before.

"I think so," Santo said carefully. "I can only speak about heart transplants because that is what I do, where the successes are great. People do very well. I mean, for the first six months there is a lot of intensive monitoring, and he has to take a lot of medicine for a very long time, some for life—"

"But will he be better-off?" Mrs. Irey asked again. "Will he have less suffering than if he says no right now?"

"There is an acute phase and a chronic phase," Santo replied. "For six months, it is a critical period. For the first couple of weeks he may even do worse; obviously, they have to cut him open. But the end result can be very good."

I shifted uncomfortably. It seemed to me that despite great advances in the field, Santo was painting a much rosier picture of organ transplantation than was warranted.

"I don't think he understands what it means," Mrs. Irey said as her husband continued to stare meditatively at the wall. "I'm not sure he can make a decision with the information that he has."

Of course, this came as no surprise to me. Hospitalized patients have a hard time properly weighing their options under the best of circumstances. In a situation like this, in which the stakes were so high and Irey was struggling just to take his next breath, how could we expect him to make such a difficult choice?

After a few more minutes, the issue still unresolved, Santo left. I stayed behind to remove the dressing on Irey's groin, where the catheter had been inserted. Irey groaned as the adhesive pulled on the trapped hairs. Slowly, methodically, I worked off the clear bandage, unwilling to give it a quick tug to end the pain.

"I know this is probably unfair, and I'm sorry to put you in this difficult position, but what would you do?" Mrs. Irey asked me.

It was a question that had been posed to me many times during my training. As I had learned, sometimes patients and their families want to hear their options and make their own decisions, but sometimes they just want doctors to tell them what to do. Of course, Irey wasn't the one asking for my advice, but there was enough uncertainty in the room to convince me that coming down strongly in favor of transplant might persuade Irey into making what I still thought was the right choice.

"I think you should have the catheterization and try to get on the transplant list," I said, looking at Irey. "Frankly, the chances that you will be offered a transplant are pretty slim. If the answer is no, at least you know you exhausted all the options. Who knows? Six months from now, you might have second thoughts. Then you might be sicker, and it will be harder to start the process all over again. Besides, it's just another catheterization—"

"Have you had it?" Irey whispered.

"It's a routine test," I replied.

"Have you had it?" he said again.

"No, I can't say I have."

"Then you can't tell me what it's like, right?"

"Fair enough," I said. Any risk or discomfort was his to bear, not mine.

Once he had extracted this admission from me, Irey's countenance softened. "I'll think about it overnight," he said. "Will you come talk with me in the morning?" I said I would. "I would like that very much," he said.

At home that night I found myself worrying about the advice I had given. Nothing about Irey's case suggested that he'd get the survival benefit that Santo had promised. How many patients like Irey, debilitated and weak, terminally ill with sarcoidosis, had been studied in transplant trials? Not many, I was willing to bet. In advising Irey to pursue a transplant, we were operating in the realm of intuition and faith. And, of course, so was he. We were pitting our faith against his.

Late the following morning I was walking through the cardiac care unit when I caught a glimpse of a patient with salt-and-pepper braids. He was in bed 10, on a ventilator, in a tangle of wires and tubes. Alarmed, I pulled aside a resident, who told me that Irey had just been brought in from the catheterization lab. A balloon-tipped catheter inflated during the procedure had apparently punctured his pulmonary artery, causing his blood pressure to drop precipitously. He had started coughing up blood and then had had a cardiac arrest on the operating table. I grabbed the chart, looking for a procedure note documenting what had happened (there was none). I paged Santo, but he did not call me back.

Then I saw Mrs. Irey. She came in, carrying a bag. I went over to her and grasped her hand, trying to think of something appropriate to say, but it escaped me. "He decided to have the procedure after you left," she said, grief-stricken. "We didn't see you this morning, so we told the other doctors."

My thoughts were like leaves fluttering in the wake of a speeding car. For the remainder of the day I tried to concentrate on my other patients, but the admonishments kept flooding in, even as I tried to hold them back. Why did you influence Irey against his better judgment? Aren't you responsible for what happened?

Irey pulled on for a couple of days, but his condition eventually spiraled downward and he died. Mrs. Irey never mentioned the conversation Santo and I had had with her husband, one that undoubtedly led to his premature death, other than to say, "He never wanted a transplant. Maybe he knew better than us."

And perhaps he did. It sometimes still amazes me, more than a decade into my medical career, how much power doctors have to affect patients' lives, for better or for worse. With that power comes a tremendous responsibility to wield it wisely, sparingly, with humility. Every patient teaches a lesson, and the lesson James Irey taught me was that a doctor's words can have terrible consequences. Though our intentions were good, the outcome to which Santo and I undoubtedly contributed was horrible. But tragedy can be a powerful lesson. Doctors often think we know better than our patients, but of course, this isn't always true.

With my course on LVADs at Columbia now concluded, I found Santo in a back room in the CCU and thanked him for letting us go on rounds with him that morning. He reminded me that I could call him any time for advice or help, and we said goodbye. In the lobby, John was waiting for me, gazing quietly at the swell of foot traffic coursing through the busy complex. As we walked to my car, I again considered the great responsibility I now carried. I was caring for some of the sickest patients in the hospital. They weren't just relying on LVADs and other high technology. They were relying on me. They were waiting for me to make decisions that would affect the rest of their and their families' lives. "I have faith in you, Dr. Jauhar," Ellen Turetz, a husky woman with short, spiky hair, had told me tearfully a few weeks prior. "I am only going to agree to the catheterization if you say so." My patients didn't know about my private struggles, and probably wouldn't care much if they did. They assumed I was practicing my craft unencumbered by mundane worries, and that is the way it should be. And yet it is impossible to disentangle your personal life from your work or you cease to be human.

The turbulence at home over money and our future was sure to die down, I told myself wishfully. Maybe our financial situation would change. Maybe Sonia would become more accepting of the academic path I had chosen. I didn't know what was going to happen, but for now I resolved not to let my personal stresses affect my work. Leaving

Columbia that day, I sorely missed being a fellow, when I had had no paternal and few familial responsibilities, when I had been able to focus almost exclusively on my work, and when the promise of a bright future had still been very much alive. Now the real world was beginning to encroach. I had hoped to keep it curtained off for as long as possible.

FIVE

Do the Right Thing

We are paid for treatment, no matter whether we cure or not.
—Vikenty Veresaev, *The Memoirs of a Physician*, 1916

A middle-aged man collapses with a heart attack. Paramedics arrive, and they do all the right things: give him an aspirin to chew, place nitroglycerin under his tongue, and administer oxygen through a face mask. Then they take him to a local hospital that doesn't perform angioplasty to open blockages in the coronary arteries. Angioplasty is the best treatment for a heart attack if performed expeditiously by experienced doctors. Instead, the man receives a clot-dissolving drug—a thrombolytic—which in his case doesn't work.

By the time the man is transferred to our hospital for angioplasty, it is too late. He is already exhibiting signs of heart failure. At this point there is little reason for us to open his blocked coronary artery because the part of his heart that is fed by the artery is already dead.

The story of this patient is one we encountered almost every day my first year at LIJ: a heart attack victim taken by ambulance to a community hospital that isn't equipped to perform angioplasty. If the man had been brought to LIJ, which has cardiac catheterization available twenty-four hours a day, the damage to his heart could have been averted, adding years to his life. But it would have required a degree of coordination and oversight that many ambulance fleets in New York and across the country lack.

We discussed many such cases at hospital meetings on how to shorten door-to-balloon (D2B) time, the time between hospital arrival and balloon angioplasty for patients having heart attacks. In 1971, Eugene Braunwald, a cardiologist at Harvard Medical School, proposed a radical hypothesis: "Time is muscle." He postulated that acute myocardial infarction is a dynamic process and that cardiac injury could be reduced by expeditious intervention. Many studies since then have demonstrated that shorter D2B time is strongly associated with survival. However, a large number of heart attack victims are still not being treated within the guideline-recommended D2B time of ninety minutes or less.

When I started as an attending, several published studies had sparked a vigorous debate over how acute heart attacks, the quintessential medical emergency, should be treated. With a million cases in the United States every year, acute heart attacks are a major public health problem, and how this debate is eventually settled is bound to have important public health implications.

When heart muscle is deprived of blood, it goes through what has been termed the ischemic cascade. Initially the muscle, stunned by a lack of oxygen, goes into a sort of hibernating state. Cells swell as sodium and calcium flow in through suddenly porous membranes, creating havoc with the cellular machinery. At this point the damage is usually reversible. But with prolonged oxygen deprivation for many minutes, cells start to die.

Studies comparing angioplasty and thrombolytic drugs have shown a clear advantage for angioplasty if it is performed by an experienced cardiologist in a high-volume catheterization lab within three hours of the onset of symptoms. Death rates after thirty days are lower by almost 50 percent. Also, angioplasty results in an open coronary artery 90 percent of the time, compared with 54 percent for thrombolytics. Moreover, angioplasty drastically reduces bleeding complications, especially in the brain.

But whether these advantages could be maintained in the real world, where delay in getting patients to catheterization labs is inevitable, had been an open question. Then a Danish study published about a year before I started at LIJ notched a major victory for angioplasty. In the study, about fifteen hundred patients who were admitted to community hospitals with acute heart attacks were randomly given immediate thrombolytic treatment or transferred by ambulance to angioplasty centers up to a hundred miles away. Even with the delays, angioplasty resulted in a 40 percent reduction in death, recurrent heart attack, or stroke after thirty days. The data were compelling enough that the study was stopped early by a data-monitoring committee.

In a related study published in *The Journal of the American Medical Association*, about five hundred patients at eleven community hospitals in Maryland and Massachusetts were randomly assigned to receive thrombolytic therapy or angioplasty. Angioplasty has traditionally been performed only at hospitals with cardiac surgeons on duty, in case there are complications, but these relatively small hospitals had none. In following up, the study found that even without surgical backup, angioplasty reduced the occurrence of heart attacks and strokes in the next six months by almost 40 percent and shortened hospital stays for the original visit by an average of a day and a half.

The net result of these studies was that LIJ was doing more outreach to try to get ambulances to bring patients with acute heart attacks directly to the hospital for angioplasty. At the same time, we were trying to reduce D2B time to less than an hour. But I quickly learned that coordinating ambulance fleets on Long Island is a gargantuan task, in part because a large number are privately owned. However, as my colleagues at hospital meetings pointed out, paramedics had already learned to take trauma and burn victims to specialized hospitals. Heart attack victims deserved no less, and many more lives were at stake.

———

My first year as an attending was packed with all sorts of such meetings. Once a month my cardiology colleagues would convene over chicken marsala and baked ziti and talk about the faculty practice plan. Rajiv would often bring up his "Queens strategy": finding a way to tap into the borough's large ethnic population—Russian, Greek, South Asian— which suffers disproportionately from diabetes and heart disease. "Out here on Long Island, we practice more preventative care," he'd say. "Patients are on the right meds. But in Queens it's a different story." He'd gripe about the hospital's refusal to accept Healthfirst and other low-paying insurance plans commonly carried by Queens patients. He'd warn that cardiologists at Jamaica Hospital, a competing facility, were already poaching patients in their emergency room who were slated for transfer to LIJ. He'd decry the clinic that LIJ had proposed to build in Queens because it was within a block of a busy internist, who might feel threatened and start referring his patients elsewhere. "As much as we hate to admit it, patients are a commodity," he once unashamedly declared when we were brainstorming about how to increase procedural volume (which would help determine his and his interventional colleagues' salaries).

For my part, I couldn't help wondering how the hospital was going to handle more patients. Where were we going to put them? The ER was already overflowing, and patients on the wards were sometimes stowed in the corridors. *Did we really need to keep putting stents into everyone?* But I kept my mouth shut. If I ever had any doubts that medicine is distinct from business, these gatherings absolved me of that notion.

The meetings multiplied, and soon I was attending hospital conferences on quality improvement and resource utilization. Published studies show wide variation in death rates between best and worst hospitals. For example, thirty-day mortality ranges from 11 to 25 percent for patients with myocardial infarction and from 7 to 20 percent for patients with congestive heart failure. The mantra at these meetings was "evidence-based medicine," which meant looking for reliable metrics, not clinical judgment or experience, to quantify performance and identify best practices. There was a kind of staleness at these meetings, a saccharine, artificial quality that permeated everything from the agenda to the muffins. People would say stuff like "We need a holistic approach that addresses the issues of variability and interdependencies" and "Let's review our program across the entire spectrum of processes," or they'd use phrases like "continuum of care" or "integrate and transform." It was corporate gobbledygook, and it never made much sense.

I discovered a tension between my dual roles as a faculty physician and a hospital employee. As a faculty physician in the Division of Cardiology, I was trying to generate more revenue for my particular section. As a hospital employee, I was trying to keep down overall hospital costs. Nowhere was this conflict more evident than in my charge to reduce the length of stay of patients hospitalized with heart failure. Like all acute care facilities, LIJ received a set payment for each admission based on the patient's diagnosis. (Such a prospective payment system for hospitals had been in operation since the early 1980s.) The longer a patient stayed in the hospital, using up a greater amount of resources, the more money the hospital stood to lose. Of course, the longer a patient stayed, the greater the likelihood of hospital-acquired infections or harm from tests and procedures, which meant that timely discharge, in most cases, was good for the hospital and patients alike.

But individual doctors, paid separately by insurers for patient visits, had little motivation to discharge patients quickly. As long as their patients were in the hospital, they could bill and be paid for each visit they made. The incentives were misaligned. The hospital was paid a fixed payment. Physicians were paid à la carte. (The incentives might have gotten aligned if hospitals had been allowed to share savings with doctors, but the law at the time prohibited any practice that might influence doctors to provide less care.) Reviewing heart failure cases, both mine and other physicians', on rounds, I frequently encountered patients getting diagnostic workups or trivial medication adjustments that could have been performed on an outpatient basis. What was keeping these patients in the hospital?

The administration did not think it was because private doctors with admitting privileges were eager to bill more. "I am not jaded enough to think that doctors are going to keep patients in an unsafe environment for an extra seventy or eighty bucks a day," Bill Remsen, a senior hospital executive, told me when we discussed it at a utilization meeting. "I really don't believe that is happening." Instead, he attributed the problem to a fragmented delivery system. "Most hospitals don't have the number of physician's assistants and nurse practitioners we do," he said. "It's a unique model: more handoffs, more confusion. Who's taking responsibility for the patient?"

However, some private doctors had a different take. One afternoon, while nursing a cup of coffee at the doctors' station on ward 7-South, I found myself discussing my administrative responsibilities with Samuel Oni, an affable Nigerian internist in private practice whose patients had some of the longest lengths of stay. When I brought up the issue of hospital stays for heart failure, he confirmed what I suspected. "I understand why hospitals want to cut down length of stay," he told me matter-of-factly. "As the length of stay goes up, they keep less money. But if I discharge a patient early, I don't get paid at all. It's okay if you have enough patients in the hospital, but if you don't, you sometimes have to drag out the stay. I don't like to do it, but sometimes you have to."

Overutilization was the gorilla in the room. Everyone could see it, but few seemed to acknowledge it was there. A fifty-year-old patient of Oni's was admitted to the hospital with shortness of breath. During his monthlong stay, which probably cost upward of $200,000, he was seen by a hematologist; an endocrinologist; a kidney specialist; a podiatrist; two cardiologists (me and another doctor, named Chaudhry, who joked, "I am just going to write, 'Agree with Jauhar'"); a cardiac electrophysi-ologist; an infectious-diseases specialist; a pulmonologist; an ear, nose, and throat specialist; a urologist; a gastroenterologist; a neurologist; a nutritionist; a general surgeon; a thoracic surgeon; and a pain specialist. The man underwent twelve procedures, including cardiac catheteriza-tion, a pacemaker implant, and a bone marrow biopsy (to work up mild chronic anemia). Every day he was in the hospital, his insurance com-pany probably got billed nearly a thousand dollars for doctor visits alone. Despite this wearying schedule, he maintained an upbeat manner, walking the corridors daily with assistance to chat with nurses and physician's assistants. When he was discharged (with only minimal improvement in his shortness of breath), follow-up visits were scheduled for him with seven specialists.

This case, in which expert consultations sprouted with little rhyme, reason, or coordination, reinforced a lesson I learned many times in my first year as an attending: In our health care system, if you have a slew of physicians and a willing patient, almost any sort of terrible excess can occur.

There are many downsides to having too many doctors on a case. Specialists' recommendations are often at cross-purposes. The kidney doctor advises "careful hydration"; the cardiologist, discontinuation of intravenous fluid. Because specialists aren't paid to confer with one an-other or coordinate care—at least as of this writing; Obamacare is look-ing to put into place payment systems that will do just this—they often leave primary attendings without a clear direction as to what to do. More important, patients don't always require specialists. Patients often have "overlap syndromes" (we used to call it aging), which cannot be com-partmentalized into individual problems and are probably best man-aged by a good general physician. When specialists are called in, they are apt to view each problem through the lens of their specific organ expertise. (Perhaps the hardest thing in medicine is to do nothing, especially when you're called for help.) Patients generally end up worse-off. I have seen it over and over again.

Oni was hardly the worst offender. He once called me about a patient who had a right lung "consolidation"—probably pneumonia, though a tumor could not be excluded—that a lung specialist had decided to biopsy. Oni wanted me to provide "cardiac clearance" for the procedure.

"Sure, I'll see him," I said, sitting in my office, checking e-mails. "How old is he?"

"Ninety-two."

I stopped what I was doing. "Ninety-two? And they want to do a biopsy?"

Oni started laughing. "What can I tell you? In my country we would leave him alone, but this is America, my friend."

Though accurate data are lacking, the overuse of health care services in this country probably costs hundreds of billions of dollars each year, out of the more than $2.5 trillion that Americans spend on health. Are we getting our money's worth? Not according to the usual measures of public health. The United States ranks forty-fifth in life expectancy, behind Bosnia and Jordan; near last in infant mortality, compared with other developed countries; and in last place in health care quality, access, and efficiency among major industrialized countries, according to the Commonwealth Fund, a health care research group.

And in the United States, regions that spend the most on health care appear to have higher mortality rates than regions that spend the least, perhaps because of increased hospitalization rates that result in more life-threatening errors and infections. It has been estimated that if the entire country spent the same as the lowest-spending regions, the Medicare program alone could save about $40 billion a year. In some cities Medicare pays more than twice per person what it pays in others. For example, Medicare spends $8,414 per person per year in Miami but only $3,341 in Minneapolis. Even within states there are huge variances. People who live in St. Cloud, Minnesota, are half as likely to undergo cardiac bypass surgery as those in Detroit Lakes, and more than twice as likely to undergo back surgery as those in Rochester. If you have gallstones and live in Wadena, you are three times more likely to have gallbladder surgery than someone who lives in Minneapolis. Among the sixty largest communities in Minnesota, there is a fourfold variation in the frequency of coronary angioplasty and a more than threefold variation in carotid surgery. The greatest variation is in a type of prostate operation, for which rates vary an astonishing sevenfold, ranging from 1.6 per 1,000 Medicare beneficiaries in Rochester to 11.6 per 1,000 in Bemidji.

We don't know exactly why these variations exist, but we do know that in regions where there are more doctors, there is more per capita utilization of doctors' services and testing, including consultations, hospitalizations, and stays in intensive care. (I am reminded of a particle collider: the more energy present, the more mass that's created.) *The Dartmouth Atlas of Health Care*, a publication of the Dartmouth Institute for Health Policy and Clinical Practice, has shown that at my hospital—hardly an outlier—Medicare beneficiaries will see on average seventeen physicians and receive more than fifty physician visits during the last six months of their lives. John Wennberg, a researcher at Dartmouth, has dubbed this supply-sensitive care—the volume of care provided is influenced by the local supply of doctors and health services—and as is by now well-known, health care expenditures don't translate into better outcomes. In fact, health outcomes in the highest-spending regions of the country may be worse. "The hospital is a great place to be when you are sick," Remsen, the senior hospital executive, told me. "But I don't want my mother in here five minutes longer than she needs to be."

Overutilization in health care is driven by many forces: "defensive" medicine by doctors trying to avoid lawsuits (unnecessary tests add an estimated $150 billion each year to the health care budget); a reluctance on the part of doctors and patients to accept diagnostic uncertainty (thus leading to more tests); lack of consensus about which treatments are effective; and the pervading belief that newer, more expensive drugs and technology are better. The most important factor, however, may be the perverse financial incentives of our current fee-for-service system. Doctors are usually reimbursed for whatever they bill. As reimbursement rates have declined to control runaway health costs, most doctors have adapted—even if subconsciously—by increasing the quantity of services. If you cut the amount of air you take in per breath, the only way to maintain ventilation is to breathe faster.

Overtesting and overconsultation have become facts of the medical profession. The culture today is to grab patients and generate volume. Internists aren't gatekeepers (as managed care advocates once envisioned) as much as ushers, escorting favored specialists onto a case with "friendly" consults, or calls for help. The probability that a visit to a physician results in a referral to another physician has nearly doubled in the past ten years, from 5 percent to more than 9 percent. Referral rates to specialists in the United States are estimated to be at least twice as high as in Great Britain. The rates reflect several aspects of American medicine: increasing specialization, the lack of time for any doctor to give to complex cases, and fear of lawsuits over not consulting an expert. At the same time, referrals are also a way for cash-strapped doctors to generate business.

Bob and Joe and Dave have an unwritten agreement to call one another when patient issues arise outside their scope of expertise. If Bob, the nephrologist, sees a patient, he finds a cardiac and a gastrointestinal issue and consults the other two specialists, and vice versa. It's not kickbacks per se, which are illegal, but there is a mutual scratching of backs. Physician-to-physician referrals are doctors loudly declaring their independence from insurers and the federal government. Insurance companies can restrict medications, tests, and payments. But they still cannot tell us whom or when we can ask for help.

When I was in training, simple referrals from internists, like patients with only mild hypertension, bothered me as a waste of time. Now that I am in practice, I have learned to welcome them. I haven't changed my mind that these referrals are probably unnecessary, and there is plenty of evidence that wasteful expert consultation is adding to health costs and creating redundant care. But as a full-fledged doctor I appreciate the business. It is hard not to view a referral as an overture from another physician, and it is equally hard not to return the favor. However, referrals can put you into a moral bind. Should you refer patients back to certain doctors—not necessarily the best doctors; sometimes even assholes who aren't particularly good with their patients—just to sustain your business?

It is a paradox of specialized medicine. Specialists are better paid than primary care physicians, but they are also less autonomous because unlike primary care physicians, they depend on other doctors for referrals. So there is tremendous pressure on specialists to keep referral sources happy, especially in doctor-saturated areas like Long Island.

In the spring of my first year at LIJ, a cardiologist named Richard Adelman sent a seventy-four-year-old woman with a leaky heart valve to the hospital for valve surgery. Adelman no longer did rounds at LIJ, so his patient, Mildred Harris, was assigned to me. Ms. Harris had few teeth and hollow cheeks and kind of gummed her words when she spoke. Besides having emphysema and diabetes, she was frail and virtually bedbound, making postoperative rehabilitation difficult. After talking to her, I decided that surgery would be too risky, so I canceled the operation, increased the dosages of her medications, and, after several days, told her I was going to send her home.

The evening before she was to be discharged, I received a call at home from a colleague asking me if I knew that my patient was scheduled to go to the operating room the following morning. Stunned, I immediately phoned the surgeon, who explained that he was being pushed to operate by Dr. Adelman, who was "pissed we got heart failure involved . . . It's a very political situation," he said apologetically. "Adelman is a big referrer."

After getting off the phone, I called Rajiv to ask him what to do. "Tell him it's unacceptable," my brother cried. "She's your patient!"

So I phoned the surgeon back. "I am the only cardiologist leaving notes," I told him politely. "I've been recommending no surgery for days."

The surgeon said he was sorry and explained that Dr. Adelman had called him directly. "My whole career I have always acted with the feeling that it's not worth it to go to town over one case," he said. "Adelman sends me a lot of business. I don't want to lose it—or your business either." He wondered if we should get a third opinion. He mentioned asking a private cardiologist he knew to rubber-stamp the decision to send Ms. Harris to surgery.

While the surgeon and I were conferring, Rajiv called me back. Inexplicably, he had changed his mind. "Just let it go," he now said. "Tell him you're a junior guy and you'll defer to whatever he says."

"Are you joking?" I said, perplexed by his change of heart.

"Look, you can't always insist on having your way," Rajiv snapped. "Sometimes you have to let people make their own mistakes."

A group of us had an urgent meeting in Rajiv's office the following morning before the operation. "Just let them do it," a colleague told me. "Medically, it may or may not be the right thing, but politically—well, if she goes back to Adelman with shortness of breath, he's going to say, 'What the fuck, we sent her over there for an operation, and those guys didn't do anything.'"

Rajiv agreed. "You did what you thought was right," he said. He reminded me that there were differences of opinion over whether mitral valve surgery was warranted in elderly patients like Mildred Harris. How could I be so sure that my judgment was correct? I told him that at the very least there should be another opinion in the chart. How could I agree to send my patient for surgery now when I had dismissed the idea in all my previous notes?

"No one is going to blame you," Rajiv said coolly. "If they take the patient to surgery without your permission, the burden is on them." He smiled slyly. "If anything, you may be subpoenaed to testify, but that's all."

When I went upstairs to talk to my patient, transporters were already there with a stretcher to take her to the OR. I asked Ms. Harris how she was feeling. "I couldn't sleep all night," she said, as the orderlies transferred her to the narrow transport gurney. "I thought you told me I could go home." I told her the decision had been changed.

Fortunately, the surgery went well, and she was discharged from the hospital after a few days. I phoned Santo Russo at Columbia to tell him about what had transpired. "This sort of thing happens all the time," he told me. "Just last week I said no to mitral valve surgery on a ninety-three-year-old. When the surgeon asked me about it, I said it was just my opinion. If they don't listen, I sign off the case. I do it in a nice way, a politically correct way. I try not to ruffle too many feathers."

"But she was high risk," I said, hoping for some reassurance. "Her symptoms were controlled with medications. Plus, she didn't want the surgery." I remembered James Irey, the patient Santo and I had forced into repeating a catheterization—with a fatal result.

"I agree with you," Santo replied. "I would have done exactly the same thing." He acknowledged the frustrations of working in a hospital where referring physicians were pushing your hand. "If you mess up relations with a referrer, you can get fired," he warned.

I told him that I had good relations with most physicians, except for maybe one or two.

"Well, if everyone likes you, then you're probably not doing a good job," he said.

———

In my first year as an attending I also sat in on meetings on how to improve the hospital's compliance with certain quality indicators. These "core measures" sprung from a general quality-improvement program called pay for performance (P4P). Employers and insurers, including Medicare, had started about a hundred such initiatives across the country. The general intent was to reward doctors for providing better care. For example, doctors received bonuses if they prescribed ACE inhibitor drugs, which reduce blood pressure, to patients with congestive heart failure. (Only about two-thirds of heart failure patients nationwide were receiving life-prolonging ACE inhibitors, a deadly oversight by busy physicians.) Hospitals got bonuses if they administered antibiotics to pneumonia patients in a timely manner. On the surface, this seemed like a good idea: reward doctors and hospitals for quality, not just quantity. It seemed like the perfect solution to the fee-for-service problem. But pay for performance, I quickly learned, could have untoward consequences.

A colleague once asked me for help in treating a patient with congestive heart failure who had just been transferred from another hospital. The patient was a charming black man in his early sixties who applied mild exasperation to virtually every remark. ("I didn't like the food, Doc. But I ate it anyways!") When I looked over his medical chart, I noticed that he was receiving an intravenous antibiotic every day. No one seemed to know why. Apparently it had been started in the emergency room at the other hospital because doctors there thought he might have pneumonia.

But he did not appear to have pneumonia or any other infection. He had no fever. His white blood cell count was normal, and he wasn't coughing up sputum. His chest X-ray did show a vague marking that could be interpreted as a pneumonic infiltrate, but given the clinical picture, that was probably just fluid in the lungs from heart failure.

I ordered the antibiotic stopped—but not in time to prevent the patient from developing a severe diarrheal infection called C. difficile colitis, often caused by antibiotics. He became dehydrated. His temperature spiked to alarming levels. His white blood cell count almost tripled. In the end, with different antibiotics, the infection was brought under control, but not before the patient had spent almost two weeks in the hospital.

The complication stemmed from the requirement from Medicare that antibiotics be administered to a pneumonia patient within six hours of arriving at the hospital. The trouble is that doctors often cannot diagnose pneumonia that quickly. You have to talk to and examine a patient, wait for blood tests and chest X-rays, and then often observe the patient over time to determine the true mechanism of disease. Under P4P, there is pressure to treat even when the diagnosis isn't firm, as was the case with this gentleman. So more and more antibiotics are being used in emergency rooms today, despite all-too-evident dangers like antibiotic-resistant bacteria and antibiotic-associated infections.

I spoke with a senior health care quality consultant about this problem at a hospital quality meeting. "We're in a difficult situation," he said. "We're introducing these things without thinking, without looking at the consequences. Doctors who wrote care guidelines never expected them to become performance measures." In other words, he explained, recommended care in certain situations had become mandated care in all situations.

The guidelines could have a chilling effect, he said. "What about hospitals that stray from the guidelines in an effort to do even better? Should they be punished for trying to innovate? Will they have to take a hit financially until performance measures catch up with current research?" Moreover, how do you correct for patient mix? Hospitals with larger catchment areas will have longer delays in treating heart attacks because of increased patient transit times. How do you adjust for these demographic factors?

To better understand the potential problems, one simply has to look at another quality-improvement program: surgical report cards. In the early 1990s, New York and Pennsylvania started publishing mortality statistics on hospitals and surgeons performing coronary bypass surgery. The purpose of these report cards was to improve the quality of cardiac surgery by pointing out deficiencies in hospitals and surgeons. The idea was that surgeons who did not measure up would be forced to improve.

Of course, surgical deaths are affected by myriad factors, so models were created to predict surgical risks and avoid penalizing surgeons who took on the most difficult cases. For example, a fifty-year-old man, otherwise healthy, who underwent coronary bypass surgery was judged to have a risk of death of about 1 percent. For a seventy-year-old on intravenous nitroglycerin with a history of heart surgery, congestive heart failure, emphysema, and other medical problems, the risk was about 20 percent or higher. Many surgeons, however, thought that the models underestimated surgical risk, particularly for the sickest patients. They criticized the models for oversimplifying heart surgery. Surgery, they argued, is a team sport, involving referring physicians, technicians, nurses, anesthesiologists, and surgeons. Many variables can affect patient outcomes that are beyond a surgeon's control. Among other things, they said, the models did not account for simple bad luck.

Surgeons began to fastidiously report—some would say overreport—medical conditions that could affect the outcome of surgery. In some New York hospitals the prevalence in surgical patients of emphysema, a condition known to increase surgical risk, increased from a few percent to more than 50 percent after report cards came into use. Some surgeons even made a habit of routinely putting patients on intravenous nitroglycerin because being on the drug conferred added risk, thus covering for a possibly poor outcome. Others tried to "hide" surgical deaths by transferring patients to hospice programs right before they died.

"It's all about the numbers," a surgeon at NYU, where I first learned about report cards during my fellowship, told me. "We have to start coding for everything, and you guys have to help us out." There would be no high-risk surgeries, he added, unless the risk was documented in detail. "If I don't operate again until next year, that's okay with me."

Despite these excesses, in the beginning there were high hopes for this quality-improvement program. In the first few years there were major gains in surgical outcomes. The most striking results were in New York State, where mortality rates for coronary bypass surgery declined a whopping 41 percent, and outcomes improved for all hospitals at all levels. In a 1994 article in *Annals of Internal Medicine*, the cardiologists Eric Topol and Robert Califf wrote that "appropriate implementation of score cards could ultimately lead to a substantial improvement in the quality of U.S. cardiovascular medicine."

But not everyone believed that report cards were causing real improvements in care. Some entertained a more disturbing possibility. Were surgeons' numbers improving because of better performance or because sicker patients were not getting the operations they needed?

In 2003, researchers at Northwestern and Stanford tried to answer this question. Using Medicare data, they studied all elderly patients in the United States who had had heart attacks or coronary bypass surgery in 1987 (before report cards were used) and 1994 (after they had taken effect). They compared New York and Pennsylvania, states with mandatory surgical report cards, with the rest of the country. They discovered a significant amount of "cherry-picking" in the states with mandatory report cards, and learned that patients generally were worse-off for it. They wrote: "Mandatory reporting mechanisms inevitably give providers the incentive to decline to treat more difficult and complicated patients," adding that "observed mortality declined as a result of a shift in incidence of surgeries toward healthier patients, not because report cards improved the outcomes of care for individuals with heart disease." Doctors agreed with these conclusions. In a survey in New York State, 63 percent of cardiac surgeons acknowledged that because of report cards, they were accepting only relatively healthy patients for heart bypass surgery. And 59 percent of cardiologists said it had become harder to find a surgeon to operate on their most severely ill patients.

(Of course, it isn't only heart surgeons who are feeling this pressure. Similar pressures are being brought to bear in other areas of medicine. For example, there is evidence that report cards on interventional cardiologists have resulted in a drop in the number of angioplasty procedures performed on very sick patients. "I said, 'Just treat her with medicine,'" an interventional cardiologist at NYU told me about a critically ill patient in shock on whom he had refused to do angioplasty. "I didn't tell them it was because I didn't want a death on the table.")

Whenever you try to dictate professional behavior, there are bound to be unintended consequences. With surgical report cards, surgeons' numbers improved not only because of better performance but also because dying patients were not getting the operations they needed. Pay for performance is likely to have similar repercussions.

For example, doctors today are being encouraged to voluntarily report to Medicare on sixteen quality indicators, including prescribing aspirin and beta-blocker drugs to patients who have suffered heart attacks and strict cholesterol and blood pressure control for diabetics. Those who perform well receive cash bonuses.

But what to do about complex patients with multiple medical problems? Half of Medicare beneficiaries over sixty-five have at least three chronic conditions. Twenty-one percent have five or more. P4P quality measures are focused on acute illness. It isn't at all clear they should be applied to elderly patients with multiple disorders who may have trouble keeping track of their medications. With P4P doling out bonuses, many doctors worry that they will feel pressured to prescribe "mandated" drugs, even to elderly patients who may not benefit, and to cherry-pick patients who can comply with the measures.

Moreover, which doctor should be held responsible for meeting the quality guidelines? Medicare patients see on average two primary care physicians in any given year and five specialists working in four different practices. Care is widely dispersed, so it is difficult to assign responsibility to one doctor. If a doctor assumes responsibility for only a minority of her patients, then there is little financial incentive to participate in P4P. If she assumes too much responsibility, she may be unfairly blamed for any lapses in quality.

Nor is it even clear that pay for performance actually results in better care, because it may end up benefiting mainly those physicians who already meet the guidelines. A few years ago, researchers at Harvard conducted a study on the impact of P4P at one of the nation's largest health plans, PacifiCare Health Systems. In 2003, PacifiCare began paying bonuses to medical groups in the Pacific Northwest if they met or exceeded ten quality targets. The researchers compared the performance of these groups with a control group on three measures of clinical quality: cervical cancer screening, mammography, and diabetes testing. For all three measures, physician groups with better performance at baseline improved the least but got the most payments (per enrollee, the maximum annual bonus was about $27). If they could collect bonuses by maintaining the status quo, what was the incentive for these doctors to improve? Another study also showed no difference in thirty-day mortality for patients hospitalized with one of four conditions—heart failure, myocardial infarction, coronary bypass surgery, or pneumonia—at 252 hospitals that participated in P4P as compared with more than 3,000 control hospitals that did not.

Several simple reforms could improve P4P. Insurers could use less stringent requirements for antibiotic delivery. For example, to minimize antibiotic misuse they could set the clock running after a diagnosis of pneumonia is made, instead of when a patient is first brought into the ER. They could also use percentile-based rankings or rolling averages over extended time periods so hospitals don't feel pressured to be at 100 percent compliance all the time. The irony is that lowering the benchmark—allowing for a bit of wiggle room—is more likely to result in proper care.

P4P not surprisingly is deeply unpopular among most American physicians. It forces them to follow certain clinical priorities—"cookbook medicine," "a rule book"—leaving them deeply dissatisfied with the loss of autonomy. Many doctors say they feel like pawns in a game being played by regulators. Instead of being allowed to exercise their professional judgments and deliver "patient-centered" care, physicians believe they are being guided on what to do with a burgeoning menu of incentive payments or strict regulations. One recently wrote online:

We as a profession are partly to blame. We allowed the insurance companies to become the intermediary between us and our patients. There was more money at first but now we suffer the "controls" they have put in place. With regulations reaching the point of insanity, the Department of Health says jump and we don't have the backbone to question or fight back. If we don't begin to take back the controls of our profession, we will become mere technicians working on the government dole.

Another wrote:

What makes this particularly difficult is that [P4P] was not imposed on us against our will. We, through our professional societies, have adopted it voluntarily. If we could simply band together and fight the external enemy who did this to us, I would have high hopes. Since we did it to ourselves, the solution will be orders of magnitude more difficult.

Doctors have seldom been rewarded for excellence, at least not in any tangible way. In medical school there are tests, board exams, and lab practicals, but once you go into clinical practice, these traditional measures fall away. Whether pay for performance can remedy this problem is still unclear. But from what I learned in my first year as an attending, it has the potential to compromise patient care in unexpected ways.

———

What then is the solution to health care overuse? One option is to hire doctors as employees and put them on a salary, as they do at the Mayo and Cleveland clinics, taking away the financial incentive to overtest. Chronically ill patients in the last two years of life cost Medicare tens of thousands of dollars less when treated at the Cleveland Clinic, where teams of doctors follow established best-practice models, than at many other medical centers. Nevertheless, many self-employed doctors recoil at the idea of institutional employment and intrusion on their decision-making authority. Another option is to use bundled payments. A major driver of overutilization is that doctors are paid piecework. There is less of an incentive to increase volume if payments are packaged (e.g., for an entire hospitalization) rather than discrete for every service. Yet another possibility is "accountable care organizations" advanced by Obamacare, in which teams of doctors would be responsible (and paid accordingly) for their patients' clinical outcomes. Of course, such a scheme would force doctors to work together and to coordinate care. Unfortunately, most doctors, notoriously independent and already smothered in paperwork, have generally performed poorly in this regard.

However, if we want to maintain the current fee-for-service system, reforms will have to focus less on payment models and more on education. Medical specialty societies recently have released lists of tests and procedures that are not beneficial to patients, including MRIs for most lower-back pain and nuclear stress tests when there are no signs of heart disease. These "appropriate-use criteria" (bolstered by "comparative effectiveness research") are essential for educating physicians and patients alike about medical services that are wasteful and should be avoided. (By employing these criteria, cardiologists have been able—or forced—to decrease their use of imaging by 20 percent.) In fact, better-informed patients might be the most potent restraint on overutilization. A large percentage of health care costs is a consequence of induced demand—that is, physicians persuading patients to consume services they would not have chosen had they been better educated. If patients were more involved in medical decision-making (admittedly not easy to put into practice in the hyperspeed that is contemporary American medicine, and also obviously at odds with regulation-driven P4P care), there would be more constraints on doctors' behavior, thus decreasing the possibility of unnecessary testing. Shared decision-making would be more likely to get patients the treatments they want, consistent with their values. This could serve as a potent check on what the doctor ordered.

Of course, health information is imperfect, and patients, ill and under duress, are often poorly equipped to understand it. (And busy doctors— our name ironically derives from the Latin word for teacher—clearly do a haphazard job of advising and instructing patients.) But even when good information is available, patients too often are passive consumers, still operating on the model of "Doctor knows best" (which many doctors admittedly encourage). For example, studies have shown that patients take little interest in the informed consent process. In a study of cataract surgery, only 4 percent of patients recalled more than two out of five risks disclosed to them by their doctors. Only a third remembered later that blindness was a potential risk.

Today roughly one out of every six dollars in America is spent on health care. If we do not succeed in controlling these costs, they will gradually crowd out other necessary societal expenditures. Improving health literacy will be critical to these efforts. Without a better understanding of what doctors are actually doing, one may end up like Dr. Oni's patient who had seventeen consultants and twelve procedures and who reinforced a further lesson I have learned many times since entering practice: When doctors are paid piecework for their services, the result too often is waste, disorganization, and overload.

SIX

Double Effect

Death is always cheaper.
—Albert L. Waldo, M.D., University Hospitals Case Medical Center

In September 2005 I received a letter from the membership and creden-
tialing committee of the American College of Cardiology informing
me that I'd been elected a fellow. The ACC, founded in 1951, is the
largest cardiological society in the United States, with nearly forty thousand members, including physicians, scientists, nurse practitioners, and
physician's assistants. The convocation was to take place in early March
at the college's annual conference in Atlanta. Fellowship in the ACC
requires completion of advanced cardiology training, passage of the cardiology boards (which I had successfully completed earlier that year),
and letters of sponsorship from other ACC fellows. I viewed it as the final step to admission into an exclusive guild.

I flew to Atlanta a couple of days before the ceremony in the spring.
The conference, a colossal affair with roughly five thousand cardiologists
in attendance from all over the world, took place at the Georgia World
Congress Center near Centennial Olympic Park. There were dozens of
talks—mostly standing room only—going on concurrently throughout
the ninety-acre complex. PowerPoint slides flashed arcane analyses on
subjects ranging from mitral valve repair to the genetics of heart failure
to stem cell therapy after myocardial infarctions. I attended one talk on
the use of left atrial size as a predictor of heart failure. How to interpret
the findings? How do you critically evaluate a study whose methodology

(Kolmogorov-Smirnov goodness-of-fit tests, proportional hazard models, propensity scores) you don't understand? I leafed through the four-hundred-page monstrosity that was the conference program book. Here was the academic-industrial complex—publication for publication's sake—in its full glory.

Between sessions I strolled through the convention center. Outside, in the muggy afternoon heat, children were playing in water geysers shooting out of the ground at Centennial Park. I passed through the gargantuan exhibit hall, where companies had set up booths to peddle their wares. At the Merck and Pfizer booths you could check your blood pressure and your serum cholesterol (through a pinprick) and receive a computerized cardiac risk profile. At the Terumo booth you could watch videotaped demonstrations on the use of robotics in the cath lab while enjoying a complimentary fresh fruit smoothie. At nearly every booth there were pretty young saleswomen passing out freebies—pens, penlights, even stethoscopes and portable music players. In one chamber a professional model, her chest covered with a flimsy white sheet, was getting an echocardiogram to demonstrate the resolution of a new ultrasound probe. Nearby, a young blond woman was receiving enhanced external counterpulsation, a noninvasive procedure sometimes performed on patients with heart failure in which pneumatic cuffs on the calves and lower and upper thighs inflate and deflate in synchrony to decrease the workload on the heart. Each compression caused her hard body to thrust suggestively, and a group of cardiologists in rumpled khakis and blazers had gathered to watch.

One session I attended was a panel debate on the safety of the heart failure drug Natrecor, whose manufacturer, Scios, still had me on its speakers' bureau and for which I was still occasionally giving paid talks. *The Journal of the American Medical Association* had just published its paper raising concerns about the drug: Did it cause kidney damage? Did it increase mortality? Sales nationwide of the billion-dollar-a-year medicine had plummeted. The tension in the room was crackling. Two cardiologists got into a shouting match discussing the merits and demerits of the drug. A Scios executive quipped that he'd been sleeping like a baby ever since the *JAMA* paper was published; he'd been waking up every few minutes to cry. It was at the end of the session that I decided the data on Natrecor were too murky to justify my continuing to speak for Scios. Within a few months I'd quit the speakers' bureau, and I never gave another paid talk on Natrecor again.

The convocation took place the following evening in a large auditorium at the Georgia Center. In a small changing room I got dressed in full academic regalia: black gown, hood, cap and tassel. The getup felt heavier than those from my previous commencements. The ceremony opened with a procession of trustees, distinguished guests, officers of the college, and newly inducted fellows. As I marched into the auditorium, I surveyed the proud, smiling faces of family members and loved ones. Old and young, they looked like so many of my patients. These were the people I was going to take care of over the next several decades. I could only hope that I would serve them well. Once we took our seats, there was the laying of a mace, a ceremonial wooden staff with a silver and gold head representing the four chambers of the heart, on a velvet cushion behind the lectern. (The mace, I later learned, is a symbol of the academic quest for truth and wisdom.) Following the presentation of numerous academic awards, the fellows-elect took a pledge to "renew and reaffirm the obligations of the Hippocratic Oath, to practice my art so as to help and to heal, so that the image of the physician will be worthy of the blessings of the afflicted and the sick."

The president-elect of the college, Dr. Steven Nissen of the Cleveland Clinic, gave the main address. He opened his speech by congratulating us on an important career milestone, "an honor that will bring you respect and admiration from your colleagues, patients, and society." However, he said, "it is an achievement that brings great responsibility and ethical burdens that will demand constant vigilance."

It was our obligation, he went on to say, to "remove the biases that stand in the way of good medicine. We need to assure that no consideration of economic self-interest will ever prevent us from giving our patients the safest, most effective, and most economically responsible health care possible." He decried the proliferation of costly imaging technologies. "The history of medicine is replete with examples of new technologies that have been rushed into practice without the evidence needed to use them wisely." From what I had seen in my short attending career, his observations were right on target.

He talked about professional integrity. "Trust is priceless," he said. "It defines the relationship between the doctor and the patient. It can be protected and nurtured and passed on to future generations. Or it can be squandered."

He said he believed that the medical profession today was too entangled with pharmaceutical companies. "In health care, where so much is at stake, even the appearance of bias can damage trust . . . Our professional journals rely on advertising to pay the bills, and our national meetings are funded by massive industry exhibitions." There were slight but clear murmurings through the audience.

He criticized contract research organizations, for-profit companies that ran large clinical trials on behalf of pharmaceutical or device companies and often steered research designs in their favor. He denounced the practice of employing ghostwriters paid by drug companies to prepare clinical trial manuscripts on behalf of academic investigators. And finally, he announced that he had begun to donate all his drug industry consulting fees to a philanthropic charity and encouraged us all to do the same. "You will sleep better at night," he said.

Listening, I couldn't help but think of my medical school graduation nearly eight years earlier in St Louis. It had fallen on my parents' thirty-third wedding anniversary, an unplanned but perfect gift. They beamed with pride as I strode into the auditorium to the tune of bagpipes. The commencement address that day was delivered by S. Bruce Dowton, a pediatrician and medical school dean, who spoke eloquently about his early dreams of becoming a doctor while growing up in the outback of Australia. "From that limited horizon," he said, "I knew nothing of the world at large, let alone the world of medicine." His words resonated with me. Not so long ago, in graduate school at Berkeley, I'd also felt as if I were in a world apart. I'd been desperate to get out of the ivory tower and join the "real world."

Dr. Dowton offered this piece of advice: "Keep a simple value system. Work out what things in life you care about, the beliefs you hold near and dear, and stick to them. You are about to go through a most tumultuous time. What are you willing to accept? What are you willing to fight for?" I'd written it down in my Palm Pilot: "Figure out a value system." It occurred to me that warm evening in Atlanta, walking out of the Georgia Center in a flowing black gown, that I'd never really done so.

In my first year as a heart failure specialist, I often took care of patients near the end of their lives. I was sometimes asked to predict how long someone was going to live. On rare occasions I was even requested to assist in someone's death. In November of that year I took care of Rose Crespo, an eighty-four-year-old woman with end-stage heart failure who told me she couldn't bear feeling short of breath any longer and pleaded with me to help her die. "Is November fifteenth a good day for you?" she asked, as though she were inviting me to dinner.

Alarmed, her daughter shot out of a chair at her bedside. "Ma, do you understand what you are saying?"

The old lady stared at her and nodded slowly. She had short, curly hair dyed brown and large spaces between her teeth. She spoke with the unvarnished bluntness of someone who has no more energy to waste on being diplomatic. "I can't take it anymore," she said. "Back and forth, back and forth to the hospital. I'd rather be dead."

I explained that I could not assist in her suicide, though I could give her morphine to relieve her suffering.

"If you were like me, you'd say the same thing, Doctor," she said ruefully. "I'm half gone. Nobody wants to bother with you when you're like this."

Not knowing what to do, I called a representative of the ethics committee, who invited me to a meeting it was having that week. It took place at seven-thirty in the morning in a small room in the basement (not far from where we had cardiology morning report). When I arrived, a dozen participants—doctors, nurses, a psychologist, two social workers, a lawyer, and a rabbi—were gathered around a conference table. They were discussing the protocol for how to rescind do-not-resuscitate orders when patients give consent to be operated on before surgical procedures. Surgeons routinely require such nullification, even for elderly or terminally ill patients who have long-standing DNR status, because of the life-threatening (and often treatable) risks associated with major surgery. "To have this kind of dialogue is difficult," a psychiatrist was saying. "How do you bring up the issue of cardiac arrest on the operating table? We may have a form for patients and physicians to sign, but let's not delude ourselves about what this form really represents"—namely, protection against medicolegal liability.

A nurse suggested that the form be amended so that along with the attending, whose responsibility this is, residents and physician's assistants could also sign the rescindment. "After all, they, not the attending, are the ones talking to the families."

"Attending physicians are not talking to the families?" a senior internist asked sharply. His voice took on a pedantic tone. "If a patient is going for a procedure, an attending physician has to sit down and talk about the risks/benefits/alternatives." (He enumerated the topics quickly, as if they all were one word.) "Are you saying this isn't happening?"

The nurse hesitated. "I'm not saying it isn't happening," she said carefully, "but attendings are rushed. They show up whenever they want. It isn't really clear what's being discussed."

"This sort of conversation has to be held with a primary care physician who understands the trajectory of the patient," a doctor declared.

"The primary care physician isn't the one doing the procedure," someone else countered.

The head of the committee, a gray-haired fellow named Frank Callahan, put up his hand to interrupt the discussion. He had on wire-rimmed spectacles and possessed the air of an English professor, down to his tweed jacket. "Historically there has been a lot of resentment from surgeons and radiologists, downstream specialists, about being ruled by upstream contracts," such as a DNR decision made in a primary care physician's office prior to a patient's being referred for a procedure, he said. "It isn't just professional ego. They're saying the guy up there doesn't understand what's going on down here." The psychiatrist started to respond, but Callahan stopped him and said that time was short and that further discussion would need to be deferred until the following meeting.

The next item on the agenda was whether a patient could refuse care on prejudicial grounds, such as a doctor's race or skin color. The lawyer on the committee argued forcefully that doctors should tell patients that they don't have a choice about who will treat them. "We should say, 'This is medically mandated, and if you want to go down the street to another facility, well, go right ahead.'" Taking the contrary viewpoint, Callahan responded that he believed that in an emergency, and if an alternative health care provider was available, it was appropriate to honor such requests. "Patient autonomy includes the right to choose who will, or will not, care for us," he said. "The doctor-patient relationship requires intimacy, and intimacy is a matter of choice." Even though the hospital would not accept directives that violated its ethical or legal obligations, he said, doctors still had a duty to sacrifice their own interests for the sake of their patients. Though I stayed quiet, I found myself agreeing with him. The bedside is not the place to wage battles for social justice.

"We have a guest this morning," Callahan announced pleasantly. He turned to me. My leg was shaking nervously. "Dr. Jauhar is our heart failure specialist and has a patient he'd like to tell us about." I nodded, looking around at the twelve or so expectant faces. Then I cleared my throat and started to present my case. I had met Rose Crespo about four weeks earlier, when she was transferred to LIJ from another hospital after an episode of acute pulmonary edema, in which her lungs rapidly filled up with fluid because of congestive heart failure. An angiogram at the first hospital showed severe and diffuse coronary artery disease that was deemed inoperable. Surgeons at LIJ agreed with this assessment, saying that the risk of death during or immediately after bypass surgery was at least 50 percent. With no invasive options, she was treated medically and discharged from our hospital after a few days. But about a week later her daughter called to tell me that her mother was again feeling short of breath. Mrs. Crespo was readmitted and again treated with intravenous drugs. Her condition improved, but when the drugs were stopped, she had another episode of pulmonary edema. This cycle was repeated several times until the day she asked me to help her die. Though initially horrified by her wish, her family had come around to supporting her decision and wanted to be in the room with her when she passed away. "It seems like what they are asking for is physician-assisted suicide," I said.

"Sounds more like euthanasia," someone said snarkily.

"She just doesn't want to suffer anymore," I said, ignoring the remark. "She doesn't want to go through another episode of pulmonary edema. She is absolutely terrified of it."

"I don't see the big ethical dilemma," the senior internist said. "Put her on a morphine drip to relieve her suffering." This would likely cause respiratory depression that would kill her within hours to days.

"But she isn't currently suffering," I replied.

"So put her on a low dose and titrate it up when she develops symptoms."

"The problem is that she can go into pulmonary edema very quickly," I said. "She could suffer for hours before her shortness of breath is brought under control, and that's in the CCU, where nurses are with her around the clock."

Callahan got up and wrote "extend life < prevent suffering" on a white board. Underneath he wrote: "Goals: hasten death (no); prevent suffering (yes)." Turning to me, he said that it was ethically justifiable to start a drug like morphine that could speed up death, as long as preventing suffering was the primary intention and hastening death was an inescapable side effect. This doctrine of "double effect" says that actions in the pursuit of a good end (symptom relief) are morally acceptable even if they result in a negative outcome (death), as long as the negative outcome is unintended and the good outcome is not a direct consequence of the negative one. It is a concept that comes from Catholic ethics. For example, as St. Thomas Aquinas argued in *Summa Theologica* in 1274, killing someone trying to harm you is justified in self-defense. The double-effect principle, Callahan went on, has been advocated by several medical societies, including the Oncology Nursing Society, which has even stated that it is unethical not to practice this way. Of course, all this raised the question of how one could start morphine in a patient who wasn't suffering at that precise moment, but I just nodded respectfully and let it go.

After the meeting was adjourned, I walked out with the psychiatrist. "It's funny," he said to me. "I've been on this ethics committee for a long time. The issues that come up are the exact same ones that we were tackling twenty years ago. I remember a young attending who was uncomfortable using morphine. The patient said, 'Take me off the ventilator, but my only worry is that I will not get enough morphine and that I will suffer.' And that is exactly what happened. That was probably fifteen years ago. Time passes, but the issues remain the same."

Later that day I put Rose Crespo on a morphine drip. With her and her family's permission, we arranged for home hospice care. But she never made it out of the hospital.

———

I witnessed so much death and dying that first year, it was sometimes hard to take. Every death challenged me to clarify my value system.

How much should I defer to a patient's wishes regarding end-of-life care? How hard should I encourage him, as I had James Irey, to make what I thought were the right choices? How to balance a patient's autonomy with the competing ethical imperatives of beneficence or social responsibility? One patient with whom all these issues seemed to converge was Joseph Cimino, a scrappy Long Islander in his late sixties whose heart failure had progressed to the point where his kidneys had nearly stopped working from lack of blood flow. Though I'd been seeing Cimino in the office for months, his disease eventually confined him to the hospital, where he spent most of his last days sitting in a chair, head resting on his palm, unable even to complete a sentence because he ran out of breath due to fluid in his lungs. He had a handsome face and thinning gray hair that I imagined had been slicked back in his younger, hipper days. Powerful intravenous drugs dripped into catheters in his arms, so edematous from congestive heart failure that a hospital ID band dug a deep furrow into his wrist. On an ultrasound his heart wasn't beating as much as twisting, trying to coax out the blood. His wife was always with him. She was an attractive woman in her early sixties with a genteel, almost Southern graciousness. They had a tender relationship, always talking to each other on visits to my office as if they were newlyweds.

Because of his age, Cimino was ineligible for a heart transplant. Though he might have qualified for a left ventricular assist device, he said he preferred death to being sustained by a machine. So he was limited to drug therapy that had become largely ineffective in his advanced disease state. "Too much fluid in the bag," he'd say, tapping on his distended belly and intermittently pausing for breath. "It's like when you're underwater . . . and you're swimming to the surface . . . because you can't breathe."

Cimino eventually developed acute kidney failure, which signified to me the end was near. Reluctantly, I told him I could put him on an intravenous drug, dobutamine, that might increase blood flow to his kidneys and possibly improve their function. It was a desperate measure; dobutamine improves cardiac performance in the short term, alleviating symptoms such as fatigue and shortness of breath, but in the long run it worsens mortality by causing deterioration in cardiac function and life-threatening arrhythmias. It is sometimes used as a palliative measure to relieve unremitting suffering. Santo Russo, my mentor at Columbia, had explained the medication this way: "Cancer doctors give drugs like chemotherapy that make people feel worse but help them live longer. We heart failure doctors give drugs like dobutamine that make them feel better but die quicker." Of course, if Cimino developed an arrhythmia from dobutamine, then his implantable defibrillator, a beeper-size device just under the skin of his chest that monitored his heartbeat, would deliver a shock, so he was protected from a sudden arrhythmic death. However, I was beginning to wonder if we shouldn't just turn off the device. Wouldn't a sudden death be preferable to a slow one drowning in his own fluids? Technology cannot change whether you are going to die, only the mode of your demise.

Lying in bed, wrapped in hospital blankets, Cimino pondered the dobutamine option. "If I can prolong my life . . . and leave the hospital . . . that would be all right," he said. "I mean, I don't want to die . . . but I don't want to put off the inevitable either."

I explained to him that patients requiring dobutamine usually had very limited life spans, a consequence of both their disease and the side effects of the drug. I brought up the option of hospice care, designed to alleviate the suffering of the terminally ill. Cimino didn't want to discuss it. "I still have hope," he said bravely, wiping the perspiration off his brow. "I know you're doing your best . . . but I still have hope."

A dobutamine drip was started that afternoon. In the evening, before leaving the hospital, I stopped by to see how he was doing. Ashen-faced, he seemed more spent than ever. "I'm waiting," he said.

"For what?" I asked.

"A miracle," he replied.

Against the odds, his kidneys did respond briefly to the new drug. Tests showed that the level of creatinine in his blood, a marker of renal dysfunction, dropped dramatically. When I informed him of this, he seemed pleased. "I don't know what to say . . . I was prepared for something else . . . to lie here and to die right here . . . and now you're telling me this." He shook his head, as though marveling at the mystery of his life. "I don't know what to do now."

I told him that there was nothing for him to do. His body would dictate how we proceeded.

His wife, her eyes moist, came over to the bedside. "If you can come

home and work on the garden and finish that model, and we could enjoy a few more weeks or months together, well, that wouldn't be so bad,
would it?" she said.

"No, I guess that would be all right," he replied, though his tone was
skeptical. "I'd like to live a little longer . . . I'd rather be alive than dead."

By the following morning, however, his demeanor had changed. "Sit
down!" he commanded when I entered the room. "If anything is going
to happen . . . I must say my piece." Stunned, I pulled up a chair, wondering what had happened. "This is too much . . . I never expected
this . . . the humiliation"—he was panting by then, as if he had just finished a race—"no matter what . . . I don't want the catheter to go back
in . . . I'll urinate on my own . . . I have that right . . ." He shook his head
in disgust. I tried to explain that the catheter was necessary to accurately
measure his urine output as well as to drain his bladder, since it was
nearly impossible for him to stand up to urinate because he was so weak,
but he stopped me. "Some of the staff . . . you wouldn't believe . . . one
aide told me . . . 'I don't like you.'" He scowled bitterly. "I mean, it's
unbelievable. This place is one step shy of"—he spit out the words—"a
prison."

Over the next few days, Cimino's condition worsened. Through my
stethoscope, his waterlogged lungs sounded like Rice Krispies in milk.
When I pressed on his belly, the veins in his neck popped out like fleshy
straws. I knew he had little time left and there wasn't much more I
could do. He would not consent to a breathing tube or dialysis, so once
he tired out or his respiratory condition worsened or his kidneys failed,
that was likely going to be the end of it.

As he entered his final days, delirium set in, waxing and waning over
his remaining time.

"Pull my pajamas down," he ordered his wife one morning. "It's hot!"
He stared angrily at me. "I was up the whole night!"

"And so was I," his wife wearily added.

"There's a smell!" he cried, pinching his nose.

Oblivious, I asked him what it was.

"I don't know . . . they give it to people when they are trapped."

"Do you smell it now?" I asked.

"Just the residue . . . oh, let me get up . . . I can't sleep." He tried to
pull himself out of bed. The oxygen mask was up on his forehead. He

pointed miserably at the IV pump, which was beeping. "This thing is going off . . . day and night."

I silenced the alarm. "Did you decide about hospice, Joe?" I asked gently.

His eyes glistened with anger. "I'm Catholic," he growled. "It's not for me to say . . . when I die."

"But you need the care," his wife said softly.

"Believe me, I know that . . . I do . . . I do." Tears started to fall from his eyes. "Just let me die . . . Might as well save the money . . . and finish me off."

His wife took me into the hallway. Her eyes were bloodshot, and she looked a mess. She had worn the same outfit for three straight days. "I'm sorry to put you in this position, Dr. Jauhar, but what would you do if it was your father?"

I had heard such questions many times as a doctor. It seemed to distill everything that patients or their loved ones wanted to know in a crisis. I had asked a similar query myself when Sonia was sick during her pregnancy. And yet it conveyed distrust, skepticism, an implication that medical care was contextual, somehow different if you loved the patient more.

"I would tell him to choose hospice," I replied without hesitation. Hospice, I explained, would focus on his comfort. A nurse would come to the home to help with the dobutamine. If Cimino developed worsening heart failure, the nurse might adjust the drug or give him Lasix or put him on a morphine drip, but she would discourage him from ever returning to the hospital.

Mrs. Cimino blinked away tears. "He's been in the hospital for three weeks," she said. "I didn't think it would take this long to go."

"Go where?" I asked stupidly.

She laughed mirthlessly. "To heaven," she said.

Cimino eventually agreed to hospice at home. By then he was staring out, glassy-eyed, gray-lipped, mouth wide open, strands of his greasy gray hair splayed out over the pillow. One morning he took my hand and placed it on his sweaty forehead. "He is taking your blessing," his wife said.

"We've been together quite a while . . . Dr. Jauhar," he rasped softly. "A whole year I've been suffering."

I asked him if he believed in an afterlife. His eyes rolled upward in an expression of resignation. "You have to believe . . . there is something . . . to keep going," he said. "Sometimes I think . . . I should keep fighting . . . but then I think . . . what's the point . . . if you're going to die anyhow?"

The room had a less tense atmosphere once palliative care was initiated. Mrs. Cimino remained composed, even in the face of her husband's impending death. "Thank you for everything you have done for him," she said the day they left. "I won't ask what religion you are, Doctor, but he has faith as a Catholic that he will live again. He is going home—" And then she broke down.

"Well, I guess that's it, then," she said after a minute, as if she had finally crossed over the shadowy boundary to acceptance. She made to leave, then turned back to me. "There was so much fluid in his belly, Doctor. If we had come earlier, would he still—"

I assured her that it would not have made a difference.

"Just look at him," she said, pointing at her husband from the doorway. "His face is so swollen." The straps of the oxygen mask were digging into his cheeks. "Why does he look like that?" I told her that his kidneys had stopped working, so any fluid going into his body was accumulating there.

"How long, Doctor?" she asked. "Will it be today or tomorrow?" I told her it would happen within a few days. "That's okay," she said, stifling a sob. "I will be with him. I will stay with him till the end."

Before Cimino was discharged home with hospice arrangements, a cardiology fellow came by and deactivated his defibrillator. At that point there was little reason to keep it on. Cimino was suffering terribly, and a sudden arrhythmia would have been a merciful event. I thought of my own grandfather's death in New Delhi in 1995, on a September morning after his eighty-third birthday. He woke up complaining of abdominal pain, which he attributed to an excess of food and Scotch the night before. After a few minutes my grandfather bellowed a loud groan and went unconscious; just like that, he was gone. He almost certainly had a massive heart attack, but that wasn't what killed him. It was the ensuing arrhythmia—the ventricular fibrillation—that prevented his heart from sustaining blood flow and life. When I talk to my mother about his death, she says she is sad that he died so suddenly. But she is thankful, too.

I often wonder how hard I should push patients with severe heart failure to get implantable defibrillators. When it comes down to it, perhaps the biggest sacrifice patients make when they get a defibrillator is the uncertainty over how they're going to die. Sure, defibrillators prevent sudden death, but they also take away the sudden death option, which for many patients has a romantic, if not practical, appeal. Defibrillators are also enormously costly, $20,000 or more each. In the United States, more than five million patients have heart failure, and half a million new cases are diagnosed each year. If even a small fraction of these patients were to receive this device, the costs could reach billions of dollars. It makes sense to implant a device in the chest of a fifty-year-old with a good life who is providing service to society, but what about a seventy-year-old debilitated by heart failure and living in a nursing home? That patient might benefit the most in terms of reducing the risk of life-threatening arrhythmias, but would also probably get less benefit in terms of "quality-adjusted life-years." Advances in medical technology, especially end-of-life treatments, raise all sorts of moral questions. Who should get care? How much is society willing to pay? Are some lives "worth" more than others? All a reminder that though medicine provides awesome technology, it does not tell us how to use it.

I received a message from Mrs. Cimino about a week later asking me to call her. I got through to her husband's voice mail. "Joseph Cimino . . . is not available. At the tone, please record your message . . ." I hung up and called an alternate number.

When I finally reached her, she said, "The hospice people have been amazing. They are doing for money what his family won't do for love. Don't get me wrong—our sons are very close to their father. But one is in Minneapolis, and the other is in the hospital with an infected foot. He wants to be here—he loves his dad—but he just can't."

She cleared her throat. "Meanwhile, I just"—I could hear her sobbing—"hate to see him suffer. Anyway, Doctor, I appreciate your call. I don't know what I was trying to achieve when I called you. Maybe there was something else we could do."

Joseph Cimino died the following morning. His wife called again the next day after he'd died. "I want to thank you for everything you've done," she said, sounding relieved. "There is no doubt in my mind that you added months to his life, and for that I will always be grateful."

I asked her if there were any lessons she had learned that she could share with me. With so many of my patients dying, it was hard not to think about my parents'—and even my own—mortality. She did not immediately respond. "Just that life is finite," she finally said. "No new lessons, I suppose." I asked if she believed in an afterlife. "No," she replied. "I'm an atheist. If there were an afterlife, he would have gotten in touch with me by now."

In the United States, patients with terminal illnesses often spend a large part of the end of their lives in the hospital. At NYU Medical Center, where I trained, patients spend nearly thirty days of their last six months inside the institution. Eighty-five percent of Americans die in a hospital or nursing facility, and a third of all health care dollars is spent on patients in their last year of life. Nearly every doctor I've talked to recognizes that this wastes precious resources and prolongs suffering. But they—I—have not been taught a different way.

Hospice is one alternative. The word "hospice" derives from the Latin word *hospes*, which means "to host" a stranger. The modern hospice movement started in 1967, when Dame Cicely Saunders, a nurse, opened St. Christopher's Hospice in London. Saunders formulated three principles for easing the process of dying: relief of physical pain, preservation of dignity, and respect for the psychological and spiritual aspects of death. In the beginning the majority of hospice patients had cancer, but in recent years cancer patients have actually been a minority. (In contrast, the number of patients in hospice with end-stage heart failure has doubled.) Today pain, nausea, and shortness of breath are properly recognized as scourges of the terminally ill and are aggressively treated. The number of American hospitals offering palliative care, which spans the spectrum from simply providing end-of-life counseling to full hospice care in the facility, has nearly doubled since 2000, growing to nearly fifteen hundred programs—that is, the majority of all hospitals. Perhaps the most surprising finding from these programs is that hospice patients live a month longer on average than similar patients who do not receive such care.

Managing end-of-life care is never straightforward. It forces a physician to recognize, and sometimes to adjust, his most fundamental professional and personal values. It often involves competing ethical imperatives—patient autonomy, physician beneficence, social justice—

that are sometimes in direct conflict. When I think of how Joe Cimino succumbed, I remember what Rose Crespo, the elderly woman with terminal heart disease who asked me to help her die, told me: "My husband said the hardest thing to do is to die; I always thought it would be easy."

SEVEN

Hatching a Plan

The bleeding always stops.
                    —Norman Shumway, cardiac surgeon, Johns Hopkins
                         University School of Medicine

Every death leaves a residue, and my patients' deaths were no exception. Like waves lapping at a shoreline, they took away as much as they left behind. Some succumbed quickly, while others lingered painfully. Heart failure was the common final pathway, yet each death was unique. And each affected me in its own way.

An old man in the CCU. A few days into his hospital stay, he whispered to me, "I am going to die here," as if letting me in on a secret. I tried to reassure him; on the scale of disease I normally treat, his case was relatively mild. But then he became sicker. His bloated legs dripped fluid from the pores, soaking his bedsheets and puddling on the tile floor. His blood pressure dropped. He became delirious. I was perplexed by the precipitous downturn. What did my patient know that I did not? After several days of keeping around-the-clock vigil, his wife could no longer bear his suffering and requested palliative care. Several hours before he died, groggy from morphine, he managed to summon a few moments of lucidity. Gripping his wife's hand, he said to her, "You're doing the right thing."

A few weeks later, a frail middle-aged woman. She told me calmly on morning rounds that she had a feeling she was going to die that day. Several hours later she complained of belly pain, and when a tube was

inserted through her nose and into her stomach, old digested blood—
resembling coffee grounds—from a gastric hemorrhage came up. Her
blood count plummeted, and within a few hours she had spiraled into
shock and multiorgan failure, even before we could get a CT scan to see
what was going on.

I don't know how these patients were seemingly able to predict
their own demise. They experienced a feeling of impending doom. Perhaps high levels of circulating adrenaline caused a reaction similar to a
panic attack; I don't know. But I quickly learned to take such intuitions
seriously.

Morbid instincts sometimes derive from other sources. In 2007, *The
New England Journal of Medicine* told the story of a cat named Oscar
who lives in a nursing home in Providence, Rhode Island, and seems to
have an uncanny sense for when elderly residents are about to die. He
goes to their rooms, curls up beside them—even those residents in whom
he has previously shown little interest—and purrs. Staff members at the
facility witnessed this behavior in the deaths of at least twenty-five patients. "This is a cat that knows death," one doctor said. "His instincts
that a patient is about to die are often more acute than the instincts of
medical professionals."

The disease always wins in the end. You don't always know how death
is going to occur—sudden arrhythmia, cardiac failure—but it is written
in the epidemiology, the statistics. The course is often tragically stereotyped; there are few surprises and no miracles. Knowing that the outcome
is ordained, that it won't change despite anything you do, can actually
sometimes be liberating. It relieves some of the pressure to follow established protocols, allows you some latitude to put more humanity into
the decision-making. You know the end result; you just don't know the
precise path. And you become humbled by the vastness and mystery of
it all.

One misty evening in December 2005, a few weeks after Mr. Cimino
died, I phoned my father. I had just finished my daily jog. I was running
a lot that winter, fighting an enveloping gloom. After exercise I felt different: more confident, relaxed, alive. In physics, kinetic energy must be
added to get a particle out of a potential energy well, and so it was with
me and running. In my office I'd sometimes run furtively in place with
the door closed before making rounds. The relief was dose dependent.

If I could manage twenty minutes, it would be six hours before I needed another fix.

The trees in Central Park that evening were glistening, as if a glaze had been applied. Leaves had collected in heavy, sodden piles; an occasional single leaf would get whisked away by the light breeze. Warblers were calling out mournfully in the distance. The anxious thudding in my chest had by then become a familiar sensation.

"Our trip to India was amazing," my father told me as I ambled down a paved path near the Great Lawn. "I was honored in so many places. Keynote lectures, plenary lectures—"

"What did you talk about?" I asked, interrupting him.

"Oh . . . biotechnology," my father replied. "Genetic enhancement. Plant breeding. But I also talked about India and how the country is doing, and what we can do to bring it to the level it deserves." My father's patriotism for his homeland was leavened with a certain ambivalence. His hatred of Western imperialism, still central to his politics in the postindependence era, was eclipsed only by his disdain for India's continuing fecklessness and third-world corruption.

"I got some bad news, though," my father quickly added. "You know my cousin Vikas? You may remember him. I couldn't see him this visit. Then I got a call. He died. Just like that."

Like most of my father's relatives, Vikas was someone I had apparently known as a child growing up in India but had no recollection of ever meeting. "That's horrible, Dad," I said, stopping momentarily.

"Yes, well . . ." His voice trailed off.

"How did he die?"

"I don't know. Must be something." For a moment he was silent. "All my friends are dying off," he went on. "I went to see someone in Delhi, a professor, a class fellow. He was dead, too. Sometimes I think I'd better clear my desk and get rid of all these papers."

The thought of my father's eventual death—that such a terrible experience was in store in my future—erased the good feeling from the run. I hesitated. "Are you afraid of dying?" I asked.

"I am not afraid, but I don't want to die," he replied without missing a beat. "Too much to do."

I had to smile. So typical of my father, I thought. Even his existential fears were rooted in real-world practicality. "So what do you think comes after?" I asked. "Do you live again or is this it?"

"As far as I am concerned, this is it," he replied grimly. "I don't know if there is anything afterward. There might be. No one knows."

The light was shrinking fast. A group of teenagers were sitting on a massive boulder, giggling and blowing smoke into the haze.

"Are you satisfied with how your life has turned out?" I asked.

"Of course!" my father replied, as if it were the most ridiculous question. "Good career, good children, a decent wife. Success is judged not by the position you reach in life but by the obstacles you have overcome. When my father died, we didn't have electricity. I studied under streetlamps. Now if I sent you the letters I get after my talks, they would amaze you."

My paternal grandfather's unexpected death when my father was thirteen years old opened a gaping hole in his life that had never been filled. Dad called it his greatest loss, one that left him rudderless and impoverished and undoubtedly contributed to his lifelong struggles and failures. When I was growing up, my father's moods determined the atmosphere. We could laugh only if he was happy. The rare gaiety in the house was usually my father's.

"But what's the point if this is all there is?" I pressed him.

"Your reputation will live on."

"But you won't know about it, so what's the point?"

"Still"—my father cleared his throat, a sign he was uncomfortable— "what you do lives on." I knew the talk wasn't going much further. Dad's intellectualism was secular. He never gave much credence to an inner metaphysical life.

Changing the subject, he asked about my job. Things were getting busier, I told him. However, money was still tight. And Sonia was still pushing me to consider private practice.

"Live within your means," my father intoned with his usual shop-worn wisdom. "And try to be happy."

"I am happy, Dad," I replied, forcing myself to sound cheery.

"Okay, that's good," he said, though he sounded skeptical. "I don't know how long your mom and I will be around. We just want to see you settled."

———

That spring the most dreaded announcement from Sonia was "We have to talk about our finances." It produced an almost instantaneous tightness in my chest, a jackhammer pounding, and for good reason. Our expenses were outpacing my hospital salary, and whatever little savings we had—wedding money, a bit saved up from our residencies—was dwindling rapidly. Sonia's father had offered financial help, but I had turned him down—at least at first—hoping to maintain the semblance of self-reliance. (And once I said no, the refusal assumed its own momentum because I felt that if I relented, he might think I had been insincere all along.) "I just want you guys to be comfortable," he said on more than one occasion, urging me to consider his tender. "I can explain the way of the world. Maybe you think it is hocus-pocus, but how can you say a song is bad if you don't listen to it?" Eventually I was forced to give in, but I hated to do it. I wanted to show that I had married Sonia despite her father's wealth, not because of it.

The arguments over money took a toll, eroding my peace of mind. I started going to work later and later and holed myself up in my office to call private cardiologists, who (perhaps self-servingly) told me there wasn't much money left in private practice anyway, unless you were willing to do unnecessary testing. My father was adamantly opposed to private practice, too. Apart from the insecurity—medical practices were failing all over the Northeast because of rising expenses and decreasing reimbursements—I'd have to give up my job, an academic title (assistant professor of medicine), and a certain degree of status. Did I really want to become another private practice grunt, overtesting, kissing ass for referrals, fighting insurers to get paid, depressed that medicine wasn't the way I'd envisioned it in medical school?

Things came to a head when my parents visited Long Island in the early summer of 2006. As usual, I drove from Manhattan to see them, this time without Sonia and Mohan. We spent the morning at a Hindu temple in Hicksville, where we attended puja. Priests with shaved heads and powdered faces were clanging bells and chanting fervently. Sanskrit syllables were shooting off their lips like bullets. I knelt on the stone floor and, for the first time in at least a year, whispered a prayer. As with many people, my relationship with God was complicated, ranging from quiet skepticism to outright atheism, with occasional forays into foul-weather faith.

Back at Rajiv's house, the mood was somber. The following day my parents were flying back to Fargo, North Dakota, where my father worked at a government agricultural research station, and we were all waiting on tenterhooks for him to bring up my career plans. In the kitchen, I rinsed out a glass and let the faucet run for a few seconds, checking the temperature of the stream with my finger. Then I filled up the tumbler, gulped down the water, and slammed the empty container on the counter. "You look so much like Dad when you do that," Rajiv said, watching me. "It's unreal how much you guys are alike."

In the living room, my parents were sitting together on the plush sofa, their dry heels propped up on the coffee table. The window blinds were closed, though it was midafternoon, and a lamp bathed the room in a depressing glow. My father was looking over some pictures of my brother's children. "What happened? You didn't have color?" he said.

"Black-and-white is prettier," my mother said scoldingly.

"I don't know," my father replied, unimpressed. "I prefer color."

I sat down to watch television. "Did I tell you that your mom went for blood tests?" my father said as I flipped through channels. "They were normal." Though my father's blood pressure was now better controlled since his stroke scare two years prior, my mother's pressure had become labile, and the medications for it were making her fatigued and her joints achy. My father had been asking why doctors couldn't fix the problem. He kept telling me and Rajiv to arrange a conference call. I had told him it wasn't that simple.

"All the tests were normal," my father repeated.

My eyes stayed glued to the television. "So what does that mean?" I said.

"The X-ray was normal, too," he added.

"So what did Dr. Williams say?"

"She said she doesn't know what's wrong. She suggested taking that medication you suggested."

"Ibuprofen."

"And she said if it doesn't get better, to go to a rheumatologist." He said the last part with a flourish, as if he had just made his point. "These doctors will shunt you back and forth. They don't have a clue what's going on. Still, she sent us a bill—"

"So what do you expect, Dad, that a doctor shouldn't get paid for seeing you?"

"That's not what I said. I just don't think that should be her primary consideration."

"What makes you think it is?"

"Many doctors are more interested in money than health! Remember that doctor who wanted to cut my foot? By God, I would have lost my foot! Now I do exercise, and I am completely cured." He looked at my mother, who stared at him blankly. "Dr. Williams gave your mom the results but didn't even write a report! She doesn't want to write anything down. She will protect herself first."

"Whatever, Dad." I was in no mood to argue against his paranoia.

"She kept us waiting for forty-five minutes."

"So?"

"That means she is an irresponsible doctor!"

"Not necessarily. I am always running late."

"She never once addressed me as Dr. Jauhar."

"So what?" I cried.

"She saw your mom for two minutes and said she needs an antidepressant. Talk to the patient first! If I had listened to her doctors, she would have been on an antidepressant ten years ago."

"How do you know you made the right choice?" I shot back angrily. "Maybe she would have had a happier ten years."

"Antidepressants will make you happy?" he said incredulously. "You think a medication will change her basic nature? Like you, she is not a happy person."

The wrangling elicited a half smile from my mother. She almost always deferred to my father in such conversations unless she felt he had crossed a line. We remained seated in silence while I seethed. My brother popped in and out. He could never sit still when my parents were around.

My father leaned forward, arms crossed. The veins in his hands were prominent. "So what is going on?" he finally said.

"With what?" I replied, feigning ignorance.

"With what? With your job!" As the patriarch of a traditional Indian family, he took it as his right to speak out about our problems, no matter how uncomfortable it made us.

"I already told you, I'm trying to figure things out."

My father leaned forward, hiking his fraying trouser bottoms over his hairy shins. "Don't do private practice," he whispered ominously. "We know so many doctors in Fargo who are having a rough time. Vijay Malhotra joined an oncology group that cheated him out of so much money. Now he is doing shiftwork in Boise on the weekends. His wife was crying to your mom."

My father's horror stories didn't carry much weight because I had heard enough of my own, about senior practitioners taking on young associates, exploiting them for cheap labor, and then firing them when they were up for partnership. I remembered a private cardiologist at a medical school mixer bragging about hiring fresh graduates, running them into the ground for two years, then letting them go and enforcing a no-compete clause in their contracts if they tried to set up offices nearby. He had done this many times.

"I have to pay my bills," I said quietly.

My father turned to my mother with a disbelieving look. "I think he is obsessed! He never used to be so money-minded."

"What is he supposed to do?" my mother cried in Hindi, rising to my defense. "He can't cover his expenses!"

My father opened his briefcase, took out a notepad, and with my input wrote down a list of outlays: rent, nursery tuition, car, insurance, parking, gas, tolls, taxi, cable, cell phone, groceries, credit card, and miscellaneous. Then he wrote down my monthly take-home pay. I was about $2,000 short a month, a deficit that Sonia's father had been covering.

"What did I tell you?" I said angrily as my father studied the paper. He shook his head in disbelief.

Rajiv, looking bored, urged us to come out with him to the backyard. My father and I followed him out the sliding glass door, up the sloping lawn, past the swimming pool, to a stone patio behind the tennis court abutting the neighboring horse farm, where we watched him shoot baskets.

"Your job is critically important," my father intoned as my brother threw up bricks. "Go to work on time, get more patients, and secure your job." His advice was essentially the opposite of what I had been planning. Instead of quitting, he thought I should work even harder and ask for a raise.

"I need more money now," I said. I felt pathetic talking about my financial troubles in front of my brother—and at his palatial home, no less—but part of me wanted him to feel sorry for me, too.

"All he does is talk about money!" my father shouted.

"I have bills to pay!"

"So send Mohan to public school!"

"That is not an option. It's one of the worst in the city."

My father shook his head in disgust. "As far as I am concerned, you can come home from work and start worrying. Worry the whole night if you want to, but in the morning go to work and do your job. If you lose your job, then it's over. It's over for you; it's over for us. Apart from the financial problem, won't you feel embarrassed? Your colleagues, your in-laws, everybody will know you were fired!"

Rajiv dribbled in for a layup.

"This is a utilitarian society," my father said. "If they need you, they will beg you. If they don't need you, they will kick you. At my job, they keep track of when I come and go."

"It's a government job! You have to clock in and out."

"Well, yes, I have to swipe my ID badge, but that is not the point. If you lose your job, we are finished. I will be the first to have a heart attack!" He hollered to a phantom audience, "He is my son! I cannot see him out on the street."

I couldn't help faintly smiling. My father was nothing if not persistent. "I'm—I don't know . . ."

"What? Tell me."

"I'm depressed."

"If you lose your job, you'll be more depressed! Things are going well—"

"Things are never going well!"

"Things are going well, and if they aren't, so what? Worrying won't help."

He was right, of course. I had made my own choices, yet I was wallowing in self-pity. What I wanted most of all was for my father to simply commiserate. But Dad never gave you what you wanted, only what he thought you needed.

"I don't enjoy—"

"If you get busy, you will enjoy. What's not to enjoy? You are a doctor!" he hollered. "You have the respect of the world!"

We walked back to the house. Head bowed, my father was deep in thought. I couldn't help thinking of the way he looked when I was ten years old, similarly stooped over his desk in our garage in Riverside,

California, reeking of rubber cement, painstakingly preparing a table for one of his research papers while exhorting me to become a doctor and never take the purely academic path he had taken. At the university, he explained, people were jealous. They stabbed you in the back. There was no job security. You might not get rewarded for your hard work. In medicine, he promised, I would have respect, wealth, and influence— all things that had eluded my talented father.

At the pool, my niece and nephew were splashing around in the water. We sat down with my sister-in-law, Vandana, who was watching them. "Why don't you and Rajiv come up with a plan?" my father implored.

"I told him I could set him up with my friend Amir Chaudhry," Rajiv said suddenly. "He is a cardiologist in private practice. Sandeep could moonlight at his office on weekends. [Many academic physicians he knew were moonlighting in private practice to supplement their salaries.] Amir told me he talked to Sandeep, but he didn't show any interest."

"Well, that seems like a good idea!" my father said, his face brightening. "Try out private practice and see if you like it."

"He will hate it," Rajiv said dismissively. "He doesn't have the mind-set for private practice."

Rajiv's operating philosophy was that doctors didn't really care how competent you were, or at least that wasn't the overriding concern when they referred patients to you. It was all about personal relationships. Rajiv understood this as well as anyone. When Dr. Singh's sister was hospitalized, Rajiv went to the CCU at 2:00 a.m. to put in a basic IV line that could have been inserted by an intern. When Dr. Kohli's father had chest pain after stepping off a plane from India, Rajiv left his family at the movie theater watching *Shrek* and went to meet him in the emergency room. "You have to learn how to play the game," Rajiv said. "Every doctor I know says I'm his best friend."

I glanced at Vandana, who was sunbathing on a recliner. "He invests a lot in these relationships, Sandeep," she said, forcing a smile. "It takes a lot of sacrifice."

"Your brother is the king of Long Island, and people still don't even know who you are!" Rajiv said disdainfully. "You've got to take these doctors out to dinner, buy them a bottle of wine, come to some of the Indian parties."

I groaned loudly.

"See, Dad," Rajiv said, as though I had just made his point. "He thinks he is better than everyone."

"Why don't you mix with people?" my father demanded angrily. "Rajiv was telling me you keep your door shut the whole day!"

"So do you," I replied lamely.

"Ha! He's comparing himself to me. I'm a scientist!"

"You're in a service profession now," Rajiv reminded me.

My brother was right. In times of stress I often regressed into the habits of my previous academic life.

"So why don't you work with this guy Chaudhry?" my father said. "He could be very helpful to you, even though he is a Pakistani—"

Now it was Rajiv's turn to groan. Dad's antipathy for Pakistan always eventually came out. His family had been caught up in brutal sectarian violence during the partition of India in 1947, when he was eight years old. He had witnessed horrific bloodshed, which left psychic wounds that bled at inopportune times.

"I have lived among Muslims, so I know what they are," my father declared. "Look at Sunnis and Shias in Iraq. Muslims killing Muslims. Only slight differences between them—they have only slightly different interpretations of Islam—but they have no hesitation to kill each other. Read the paper! A Hindu will think twenty times before killing anybody. It is the biggest tragedy for India that we have Pakistan as our neighbor. The worst neighbor one could have."

"Dad, you're not helping," Rajiv said.

"What am I saying?" my father said defensively. "Keep good relations with Chaudhry because you need the work. But I would not expect too much from him. I cannot generalize, but Pakistanis are not as broad-minded as we are. He'll be stingy and mean and . . ." He started losing momentum. "Anyway, it's okay, you need him, you need another source of income. And Sonia was telling me she is going to work, too."

"That's what she says," I said skeptically. She'd been promising to find a job for several months now. "We'll see."

"I know, Bubboo, but remember your job at LIJ is critically important. You cannot work for Dr. Chaudhry at the cost of that job." His face softened. He looked tired. "Life is not a bed of roses, my son. You have so much going for you. I meet people all the time who say, 'Oh, you are Jauhar, you write for *The New York Times*.' I say, 'No, that is my son,' but I feel so proud. Don't burn your blood. Life is too short."

In the early evening, my parents and my brother walked me to the circular drive. The sun was starting to set. Mosquitoes were buzzing rapaciously around me, and violet impatiens were blooming brightly on the stoop. My parents were supposed to fly out the following day. I felt a vague longing for them to stay. My heart ached when I remembered how Dad used to return from research conferences with a bag of airplane peanuts or a couple of Brach's candies for his kids.

When he hugged me, my lips trembled. I cleared my throat. Then, before I could get into the car, I started sobbing. My mother started crying, too.

"What is it? What's the matter?" my father said, feigning alarm. Then he started laughing. His reaction was the exact inverse of mine. The more I bawled, the more he laughed, as though he could assuage my melancholy with his fake jolliness. "What is it, Bubboo?" he said affectionately, patting my head as though I were eight years old again. I thought of how he would be dead one day, and it made me cry even harder.

Between sobs, my mother said in Hindi, "Just looking at him makes me so sad."

I wasn't sure why I was crying. In human physiology there is the concept of referred pain, in which a painful sensation is perceived to be in a different place from where the injury actually has occurred, and so it is with emotions, too. It wasn't just about my job or financial frustrations but something else: my relationship with my father, how he was with me—or perhaps just how he was. He had been so detached while I was growing up. I had always been desperate for his approval. Once, in sixth grade, after I'd done something to annoy him, he complained to my mother: "He used to be such a good kid. He used to listen, eat fruits." Tearfully, I had told him that I did still eat fruit, that sometimes I stopped in the grove after school and picked an orange. That upset him even more. "You're eating the fruit from that orchard! It has pesticide on it. You could die if you eat that fruit!" My mother got on my case, too: "It is poison, son. You'll get sick!" My pathetic attempts at regaining my father's good graces usually failed miserably.

Before I drove away, my father offered some more advice: "Now that we have come up with a plan, don't rehash everything. Keep yourself busy. An idle brain is the devil's workshop, so keep as busy as possible. And when you go to work, work! The job has to be your first priority. And move to Long Island to be closer to your job."

The advice had a familiar ring, and I felt comforted. I started to back out of the driveway, but he stopped me.

"Take care of your health, too. Eat fruits. Exercise regularly. If you are healthy, you can face problems much better. Save money, too, as much as you possibly can. You will need money for good times and for bad. And make some friends, Sandeep. You have no friends. I was thinking, Neeta's husband, what's his name, Jeff?"

"Fred."

"Yes. Why don't you invite him over for a drink? Make him your friend. He is a doctor, too. The problem is, you are not tactful like Rajiv."

I nodded. Salty mucus ran over my upper lip.

"If you need to talk, you can call me anytime," my father said. "Midnight, three o'clock, one o'clock, anytime. I am there for you. Always keep busy. It is not falling in water but staying there that drowns a man. An idle brain—"

"I heard it, Dad, I heard it," I said, raising the window. I started to drive away.

My father raised his hand in salute. On his face was an expression I had never seen before, somewhere between smile and scorn—or perhaps disgust. "Don't worry," I heard him say as I drove off. "Worrying doesn't help. And please call us because we will constantly be worried."

Rajiv called Dr. Chaudhry on my behalf that night. We made an appointment to meet the following week.

EIGHT

Pact

Go after exactly what you want, not what you want. For you never get
anything but the things that you exactly wanted.

—Alan Gregg, twentieth-century physician

Amir Chaudhry's main office was in a gray building standing on concrete pillars in a leafy middle-class suburb on Long Island with narrow
streets and old clapboard houses that had a certain weatherworn charm.
Just down the road were a strip mall and, beyond it, the local high school,
where a sign out front announced the weekend's sporting events. My
appointment was at one o'clock, but Chaudhry had called me that
morning to ask me to come a bit early. He had a full roster of outpatients, and once he was done at the office he had to make rounds at two
hospitals.

The waiting room on the second floor was packed. I checked in at
the front desk and took a seat among the throng of mostly Indian and
Pakistani patients talking on cell phones or tending to their infants. His
assistant soon called me in. She led me down a narrow corridor to
Chaudhry's chamber. Manila folders were stacked in tall piles on an elegant cherrywood desk. On the walls were framed certificates from hospitals in Karachi and Queens. On the far side of the room was a poster
of an illuminated lighthouse that read "Success doesn't come to you.
You go to it."

After about five minutes, Chaudhry entered. He greeted me warmly
and asked me to sit down. A short, balding Pakistani in his mid-forties,

he had huge red ears, gold wire-framed glasses, and a white coat embroidered with the words "We Care." He sank into a leather chair behind his desk, swiveling sideways to face a bureau with pictures of his four children. The piles of folders hid most of his body, save for his head and shoes, expensive Hugo Boss loafers. We made small talk for a couple of minutes—when was I going to move to Long Island?—but I could tell he was eager to get to the matter at hand.

He started off by saying that he had discussed my situation with Rajiv, whom he considered like a brother, and that he was glad to help. But first he wanted to tell me a little about his practice.

I nodded, feeling abashed at being so exposed.

He had been working as a cardiologist for five years, mostly as a solo practitioner. About a year prior he had tried partnering with another cardiologist, but that relationship had not worked out.

"I needed a second office," he explained. "I was losing patients from the hospital who did not want to come to the South Shore, so I thought if I had an office in Queens, patients would follow me and my days would be totally busy."

"Your days weren't busy enough already?" I asked. It came out like a challenge, which I had not intended.

Chaudhry smiled wanly. "A year ago I was not as busy as I am now," he replied. "Just look at my eyes." They were bloodshot. "This week I have slept only about six hours a night. See these piles?" He pointed to the folders on his desk. "These are echos"—heart ultrasounds—"I still have to finish."

There must have been hundreds. Chaudhry told me the discs were provided by a mobile imaging company, which had arrangements with local internists to perform echocardiograms in their offices. Insurers that covered the imaging paid the company, and the company paid rent to the internists to station their own employees on the premises. "I don't know what the exact setup is," he said quickly. "I am just collecting a fee to read the study."

I shifted in my chair. The phone rang. He picked it up. "Patient is here? Okay, two minutes."

He turned back to me. "I wanted to talk to you before we make a schedule so you will understand about private practice. See, Sandeep, you are in a different world at LIJ. You don't think about the business side of things." I nodded agreeably. "But don't worry," he quickly added. "You will soon get the hang of it."

The arrangement he had in mind was the following: He wanted me to take over his emergency room calls at LIJ (so-called doc-of-the-day), which meant that once a week I would be admitting ER patients who required cardiac monitoring but did not already have a cardiologist. Chaudhry would collect the insurance payments for my admissions and pay me a flat fee (which would be in addition to my regular LIJ income). He said he was trying to transition out of hospital work altogether. "You don't make much money in the hospital," he said dismissively. "If I see ten inpatients, that's about six hundred dollars. But if I sit in the office, I can stay in one place, get the echo done—that's three hundred and fifty dollars—get a stress test—that's eight hundred dollars. Plus, what is the liability in the office? Office patients are stable. They are not going to crash on you."

It all seemed pretty mercenary, but from what I'd heard about Chaudhry and his practice, I wasn't surprised. At that point I viewed working with Chaudhry as a necessary but short-term evil. I simply nodded and allowed him to proceed.

In addition to his inpatient work, Chaudhry wanted me to do weekend shifts in various satellite offices he had set up. I would supervise nuclear stress tests, see patients, and maybe read a few echos. He predicted the shift would run until midafternoon.

"Ali, my physician's assistant, will be with you," he said. "He will see patients, too, but you must stick your head in and say hello. Patients want to see you, not a PA. If they are unhappy, they go back and complain to their primary care physician."

He did not have to explain that that would be a bad thing.

"The whole thing is screwed up because we are dependent on primary care doctors," he went on. "They are jealous that why should cardiologists make all the money. They see a patient for fifty dollars, so they are not happy that you or I can get eight hundred dollars for a stress test. So instead of referring their patients to us for echos, they rent out their offices to echo companies, or they hire cardiologists to work directly with them and pay them a fixed fee. That is how the whole thing gets corrupted. Some people are just too greedy about these things."

I glanced at the piles of echos but didn't say anything. He seemed unaware of the irony, that he was complaining about the greed and corruptibility of other physicians.

He mentioned an internist who had been referring patients to him. "Last month he sent me only one patient. And this month only one patient."

Unsure of what he was driving at, I nodded hesitantly.

"So I understand something must have happened," he said.

"Like what?" I asked.

He threw up his hands, exasperated by my obliviousness. "He met someone else! He developed a relationship with another cardiologist."

I couldn't help but smile at the overwrought response, with its connotations of a romantic breakup. Again the phone was ringing, but this time he ignored it. "I tell you, these primary care doctors are crooks. They will tell you that you are good, you are the best, but then they make a deal with somebody else. Top Medical Group—you know them? Singh, Doshi, Lieberman—they were sending me one hundred percent of their patients. Now for last one year I have not seen a single patient from them. Even patients who want to see me, they do not get a referral."

"Why?"

"Because backroom all sorts of things are going on. Everybody is cutting corners."

"Kickbacks?" I said, vaguely excited by the turn in the conversation.

"In slang you can say 'kickbacks,' but they have some form of contract, paying sham office rent, something. They are not doing anything illegal, but it amounts to the same thing." He laughed. "See, Sandeep, you are a good person, a good physician, good at heart. But you are naive about private practice."

Kickbacks in medicine have long been regarded as improper. The Canadian Medical Association has declared that "trafficking in patients," implied by "secret commissions" for patient referrals, is "entirely unethical." However, to judge by recent fraud investigations, kickbacks are becoming more common. In 2006 the Tenet Healthcare Corporation, based in Dallas, agreed to pay $21 million to settle a whistle-blower lawsuit asserting that a hospital it owned in San Diego had paid kickbacks for referrals. (Tenet did not admit wrongdoing.) That same year, a New Jersey teaching hospital was investigated for giving sham salaries to community doctors in a reported attempt to increase the number of referrals to its cardiac surgery program. Two cardiologists pleaded guilty to federal fraud charges.

Chaudhry finally picked up the phone. He told the caller he needed a few more minutes.

"I had a relationship with the internist Neha Bansal for two and a half years," he said to me, sounding more and more like a spurned lover. "Me and your brother were with her uncle in the CCU till two in the morning on Ramadan. I left the mosque in the middle of prayers. Two months later, she kicked me out of her office. Not because her uncle died, no, but because she developed a connection with somebody else."

He waited for a response, but I said nothing.

"I told her, 'Send me your patients. I can do a better echo. I will pay you the same rent.' But still she kicked me out."

"Why?"

"Probably she thought I am stepping on her toe, advising her to do business with me and not with the other guy. See, Sandeep, society is corrupt. Remember that heart failure patient I sent you? Patricia—I forget her name. She was so sick. I didn't worry that I am losing one hundred dollars to Sandeep. She got better care from you, so it made me feel good. Saving life, getting patients better, is also a part of medicine. But if you try to explain this to some of these doctors, you will not be able to make a living."

He stood up and closed the window blinds, blocking out the swath of sunlight cutting across the desk. "Come, let me show you the office," he said. We walked through the warren, past an alcove where patients in salwar kameez and sneakers were waiting for their exercise stress tests, past three exam rooms and a room with a treadmill, to a procedure room, where nuclear scans were performed. His setup was not unusual for a private cardiologist. Though doctors are prohibited from referring patients to imaging centers in which they have a financial interest, they are allowed to operate that equipment in their offices, where study results are more readily available to them. "We just got this new camera," he said proudly, pointing to a solid-state instrument about the size of a child's car seat. The monthly lease, he told me, was $4,500. He broke down the other monthly costs of doing stress tests: treadmill lease, $400; office space, $1,000; technician's fee, $1,800; nurse's fee, $1,000; and miscellaneous expenses of $200.

"Now, say I get eight hundred fifty dollars per stress test," he said. (Reimbursement for these tests has since been cut by almost 50 percent because of an explosion in medical imaging and in an effort to prevent abuses.) "Then I have to do at least ten tests a month just to cover the costs, no profit going into my pocket."

"So," I said, "there's pressure on you to do more than ten stress tests a month, whether the patients need it or not."

He shrugged and said, "That is what I have to do to break even."

A monitoring board, he added, had to authorize the procedures. "Nuclear is such an expensive test. A person sitting at the company decides whether you need it or not. They deny you for whatever XYZ garbage reason. If you make one mistake—wrong number on the address, bill not sent on time, preauthorization not taken on time, anything—you get denied. If you don't resubmit within ninety days, they say time expired. Now, let's say there are even a couple of denials a month. Multiply that by all the physicians in the plan and you see how much money doctors are not getting paid. We lost so much money the first few months that now we don't schedule any tests until authorization is obtained and confirmed."

I asked him who did that.

"A clerk, the office manager, and my wife. And I myself also check."

We returned to his office. The stacks of folders now seemed even taller. "People complain that we are overtesting," he said, gesturing at the clutter. "But if a patient comes to your office and asks if she has mitral valve prolapse"—a common abnormality—"what will you do? On physical exam you will never find it, so what will you do? If she goes for a procedure and gets infective endocarditis, your career is over, so what will you do?" I stared at him blankly. He threw up his hands. "You will get an echo, right? She is already asking, 'Do you think I have mitral valve prolapse?'" He said it mockingly, with affected high-pitched worry. "People are going on the Internet; then they come to your office and say, 'I have good insurance. I pay my premiums. Why can't I have this test?'"

I asked him what percentage of echos performed in private practice was necessary for patient care. He thought about it for a moment. "About fifty-fifty," he finally replied.

"When I started in practice, I really wanted to do the right thing," he said with a touch of regret. (At that moment he reminded me of

Mr. Kurtz in Conrad's *Heart of Darkness*.) "A young woman would come in with palpitations. I'd tell her she was fine. But then I realized that she would just go down the street to another physician, and he would order all the tests anyway: echocardiogram, stress test, Holter monitor—stuff she didn't really need. Then she'd go around and tell her friends what a great doctor—a thorough doctor—the other cardiologist was." He laughed dolefully, obviously resigned to the culture in which he found himself. "I tried to practice ethical medicine, but it didn't pay, from both a financial and a reputation standpoint."

Before leaving the office, I asked him how we were going to divide the outpatient revenue. "My overhead is fifty percent, but because you are Rajiv's brother, I will say forty percent for you," he said. "The billing company keeps seven percent. The remaining fifty-three cents, how do you want to distribute?"

"You tell me," I replied.

"For office visits, how about seventy-thirty for me? When you order echos and nuclears, we will stick with the same number."

"That's fine," I said, just wanting to leave. I quickly calculated. I'd be keeping about fifteen cents of every dollar I earned, but it would still probably be enough to cover the deficit I was running at home.

"Okay, that's it," he said, looking pleased. I stood up. He came around the desk and put his hand on my shoulder. "I will send you a contract in the mail. We will see how it goes for a few months. Just remember, we need to keep the business going." Then he quickly added, "But I will never tell you how to practice in my office."

PART II

ASPERITY

NINE

Stress Test

"Up till now," he said, "life has seemed an endless upward slope, with
nothing but the distant horizon in view. Now suddenly I seem to have
reached the crest of the hill, and there stretching ahead is the downward slope with the end of the road in sight."

—Elliott Jaques, "Death and the Midlife Crisis,"
International Journal of Psychoanalysis, 1965

It took a year to process all the paperwork, but in the fall of 2007 I
finally received permission from LIJ to start moonlighting in Amir
Chaudhry's practice. The hospital agreed to extend my existing malpractice policy to cover my work at Chaudhry's office; that meant I didn't
have to purchase new insurance for the moonlighting work (roughly
$17,000 a year, prohibitively expensive given the $30,000 or so per year I
was expecting to earn). My regular weeks at the hospital were already
long—for months I'd been coming home at eight o'clock to a stack of
bills and a sleeping three-year-old—and now I was staying up past midnight to read Chaudhry's echos and working on weekends, too. As Rajiv
had predicted, I hated the work—the assembly line of unsuspecting patients, the constant subtle pressure to order nuclear stress tests and other
revenue-generating procedures—but I didn't know what else to do. Our
expenses were growing, Sonia was already talking about having another
baby, and the moonlighting, if nothing else, quenched any talk of my
going into private practice full-time—at least temporarily. The benefits
were obvious, but that didn't make me despise the work any less. It felt

as if I were being carried in a canoe down frothing rapids, and any attempt to paddle out of them was in vain.

Saturday mornings now evoked a vague melancholy, nostalgia for a time in my life—perhaps before I got married, certainly before Mohan came along—when things were less settled and I was free to chart my own course. Images from my childhood regularly popped into my head: for example, my father getting ready for work, brushing his teeth, clearing his throat, spitting loudly into the sink. I used to feel so sorry for him, for his regimented life, for his failure to relax the constraints that bound him. And now, how were things any different for me?

There was another recurring vision: Dad running after us with a shoe. He had just received his termination letter from the university, and his patience with our sibling catfighting had come to an end. We were sprinting from the living room to the kitchen, just one step ahead of my father, when Rajiv, who was fourteen, cut me off, allowing my father to grab hold of me. He hit me several times hard on the face, stinging slaps on wet cheeks. I was sobbing hysterically, not from the pain but because I had disappointed him. Rajiv flew out the front door, escaping the brunt of the anger but also waiving any right to the near-tearful apology when my father came to his senses or to my mother's tortured explanation that my father was under a lot of stress.

Chaudhry had me going to various satellite offices, where I would see up to twenty patients in a morning while reading echocardiograms and supervising exercise stress tests in between. In exercise stress testing, patients typically run on a treadmill, have a radioactive chemical injected into their veins, and then get pictures of their heart taken with a special nuclear camera to determine if there are blockages in the coronary arteries. If there are obstructions causing ischemia—a reduction in blood flow to the heart—there will consequently be less nuclear tracer uptake in certain portions of the exercising muscle, which shows up as a paucity of radioactive signals in pictures of the heart under stress. Stress testing allows doctors to determine a patient's exertional capacity, evaluate chest pain, and obtain objective evidence of myocardial ischemia. A variety of exercise protocols are available, with graded increases in speed and incline on a treadmill being the most widely used.

Chaudhry had been instructed by LIJ to pay me a fixed hourly wage, regardless of how many patients I saw or tests I performed—

apparently to remove any financial incentive for me to order unnecessary procedures—a stipulation to which he readily agreed, as it allowed him to keep even more of the revenue. I'd sometimes wake up thinking he was taking advantage of me. I'd work myself into a lather before the day had even begun. It was a loose thread in the fabric of my mind, but I couldn't let it go, and the more I tugged on it, the longer it grew. Perhaps this is how Dad felt about Dr. Yermanos, I often thought, the colleague with whom he'd had a long-running and self-destructive feud. But no one wanted to hear my complaints—not Sonia, who was busy preparing for her internal medicine board exams, and least of all Rajiv, who believed he had gambled his friendship to set up the whole thing.

I always felt as if I were selling my soul when I went to Chaudhry's Queens office, a white-shingled colonial in a middle-class neighborhood dotted with Chinese take-out places and storefronts advertising cheap divorces. Inside the building, grimy green carpeting led down a dilapidated corridor, past thin-walled exam rooms and a closet-size toilet, to the nuclear stress lab, where the radioactive isotopes for heart imaging were stored. (I often worried about what would happen if I waved a Geiger counter in there. Best not to know.) I worked with a spare weekend crew: Denis, an overweight Nigerian nuclear technician; Samantha, a pretty twenty-something West Indian office manager with a perpetually cheery disposition; Ali, a physician's assistant who had a penchant for telling fictitious stories about women he'd laid; Eva, a young Lithuanian sonographer with bright pink toenails and a prominent serpent tattoo on her lower back; and Malik, an aging Pakistani doctor who ran the treadmill.

The patients we saw often already had cardiologists but inexplicably had been instructed by their primary physicians to stop seeing those doctors and start seeing us. Queens was like a black market, where the currency was referrals and poorly health-literate patients were traded back and forth like commodities. Of course, we were paid for each patient we saw in the office—so-called evaluation and management (E&M) fees—but the primary business objective was to order a procedure. A stress test could get you $800, ten times the average E&M payment. I always made a point to ask patients if they had previously undergone stress testing, and they usually had—about six months before, someplace in Queens—but they had almost always forgotten where, and they almost never knew the results. An electronic medical record would have been very useful. So much testing could have been avoided. (But with already slim margins, no doctor I knew was looking to invest $30,000 in a system that could possibly cut revenue.) However, without electronic charts, the easiest thing—the most practical thing—was to repeat the test.

We did stress tests on at least three-quarters of the patients who came in. There is almost no evidence to recommend stress testing in patients with recent coronary stenting, but Chaudhry's staff did this routinely. There is no evidence that stress testing for coronary artery disease in intermediate-risk adults without symptoms is beneficial, but this was the bulk of the practice. The more tests you perform in a lower-risk population, the more falsely abnormal results you are going to get, leading to further testing and potentially harmful invasive studies like cardiac catheterization. (This is often referred to as an example of Bayesian probability: a positive test result is more likely to be false as the prevalence of a disease drops in the population being studied.) "Thank you for referring your patient for cardiac catheterization after a positive stress test" read a typical letter from an interventional cardiologist to Dr. Chaudhry. "Cardiac cath revealed normal coronaries and normal left ventricular function. The patient was reassured and discharged home under your care." It was a self-sustaining machine, and a whole network of doctors benefited from it; it was our lifeblood.

Every office procedure generated a follow-up visit so patients could discuss their results. However, a lot of the time the echos or EKG monitors hadn't even been read—more often than not you could find insurance documents or preauthorization forms but not the test results you were looking for—so you'd have to scramble to interpret them on the spot or promise a phone call or set up another visit. Once, I asked a patient who'd had a normal stress test if she was still having chest pains, and she told me she didn't have chest pains—she'd never had chest pains!—even though it was written all over the chart. In residency, if you didn't want to be bothered to admit a patient with chest pain in the middle of the night when you wanted to sleep, you'd push hard on her ribs and ask if it hurt, and if she said yes, you'd diagnose benign musculoskeletal pain and turn away the admission. In medicine we so often choose to see what we want to see, and Chaudhry's staff was no different. There were few checks and balances. You could document whatever you wanted. Anything to justify a procedure.

I rationalized my involvement by telling myself that I was carrying out orders, that I myself hadn't requested the unnecessary tests, that I could limit testing in any new patients I evaluated, and that if I quit, Chaudhry would just get somebody else. Still, I felt tainted. I worried about what my colleagues would say if they knew what I was doing. Did the fact that I had opted to work with Chaudhry mean that I was less upstanding than I gave myself credit for? Or that he was simply more honest about the realities of medicine?

One typical Saturday morning I pulled myself out of bed just after eight o'clock, the hour I was supposed to have arrived at Chaudhry's office. Lead-footed, I stepped groggily to the bathroom. A morass of cotton filled my head. At the mirror I rubbed the detritus of sleep from my eyes. They were bloodshot.

"Sandeep, where are Mohan's shin guards?"

I splashed cold water on my face.

"Sandeep! Where are his shin guards?"

I applied a dab of toothpaste.

"Sandeep!"

"I don't know," I mumbled.

"He can't play soccer without them."

"I don't know where they are."

"But you brought him back last time." I started to brush my teeth. "Where did you put them?" I squinted at my reflection. "Sandeep!"

"I don't know. He just took them off. You'll find them."

"But where!"

By the time I got into my car, it was almost eight-thirty, and I was already a half hour late. Traffic on the Grand Central was light; debris jutted out of dirty snow piles on the side of the road. Speeding to Queens on that lonely stretch of freeway, I felt ashamed about how I had lost my temper with Sonia the previous night. The irritations were accumulating. I was juggling too many different things. Spending so little time with my son was gnawing at me. My obligations were like the concrete embankments along the expressway, preventing me from getting off.

"Good morning, Dr. Jauhar," Samantha said cheerfully when, having nearly slipped on the front steps, I arrived at 9:00 a.m. Pulling off my coat, I nodded a perfunctory greeting and brushed past her to my office. "I'll tell Malik he can get started," she called after me. "There are already four patients waiting to see you."

On my desk were stacks of lab results and radiology reports to review and a few echos to interpret. I set them aside and brought in the first patient.

He was a thin black man smelling of liquor and cigarettes who said he'd been instructed to see me prior to undergoing a hip operation. Before he even sat down, he told me he wasn't going to have a stress test. He had had one a few years back, some outfit in Forest Hills, but he couldn't recall where exactly. "Just clear me so I can have my surgery," he said.

"That's not how it works," I replied, logging on to the computer.

"Oh, so you tell me how it works," he retorted.

"You're going to have to wait till I do my evaluation," I said. "I don't want you to waste your time or mine by telling me how to do my job."

"I'm not doing no stress test," he insisted.

"That's fine," I said, raising my hand to quiet him. "I don't care."

"Well, I know you don't care. What do you think I am, stupid?"

He had been a construction worker but had been unable to work in recent months because of pain in his hip. The hip surgery had been put off because of his drinking, which had caused abnormalities in his blood count. I asked him if he had brought a list of his medications. He nodded. We stared at each other for a moment. "So let me see it," I snapped. He laughed, then reached into his bag and pulled out a large Ziploc bag with twelve bottles. I entered the drugs into the computer. I asked him if he was taking any other prescription drugs. He said he had left a few at home.

"Are you taking a beta-blocker?"

"Yes."

"Which one?"

"I don't know."

"Is it atenolol?"

"Yes."

"Or Toprol?"

"Uh, yes."

"Coreg?"

"Yes."

"You were taking all three?"

"I think so."

"That's impossible. They're all the same type of drug."

He waved his hands dismissively. "I don't have no problem with my medicine."

"Well, were you even taking a beta-blocker?" I said. If not, I would need to start one to minimize the risk of the operation.

"I don't know. Every doctor I go to changes my medicine."

"Who is your primary doctor?"

"He's on the side."

"Which side?"

"That side." He pointed at the back wall.

"What's his name?"

"Singh . . . Singh something."

I sighed. He smiled, apparently finding our jousting amusing. "I can't believe I'm paying for this kind of abuse," he said.

"I'm not getting paid enough to listen to you," I retorted, though I was beginning to like him.

"Listen, kid—"

"Who you calling 'kid'? I'm almost forty."

"Wow, you look good."

"Well, I don't drink."

"Oh, when did you quit?" I shot him a look. He smiled impishly. "Oh, you mean you never drank!"

And so it went on for several more minutes. After inputting his history into the computer, I told him I needed to examine him. He got up on a vinyl exam table covered with protective paper bearing a drug company logo. I asked him to hold his breath so I could listen to his heartbeat. He continued to breathe rapidly. Through the wall I could hear the thump-thump-thump of heavy steps on the treadmill. "Walk, walk," I heard Malik bark. "Stand straight . . . Don't look down . . . Look up! . . . Walk!" I pictured some overweight Indian *bhainji* in a sari and sneakers trying to keep up with the moving floor.

"Do you ever feel short of breath?" I asked my patient, putting away my stethoscope.

"Sometimes."

"What about over the past twenty-four hours?"

"Well, I breathe through my mouth."

"But do you get short of breath?"

"Sometimes."

"What about in the past twenty-four hours?"

"Like I said, I mostly breathe through my mouth."

"Okay, let's try one more time. Do you get short of breath?"

"Yes!"

"What about in the past twenty-four hours?"

"No, I'm okay."

A short while later I was recording my exam when Denis, the technician, walked in and asked me to come to the procedure room. "Patient is not feeling well," he said drily.

I took a minute to finish up with my patient. I told him that because of his cardiac risk factors and my inability to assess his exercise capacity resulting from his hip pain, I was going to order a stress test with the drug Persantine, used to evaluate the hearts of patients who are unable to exercise. Once it was completed and interpreted, and assuming it was normal, I would write a note to his internist clearing him for the surgery. To my surprise, my reasoning seemed to satisfy him, because he immediately agreed to this plan. I told him to see Samantha at the front desk to make the arrangements. Then I hurried across the hall to the treadmill room. An old lady was sitting on an exam table, eyes closed, teetering precariously. She had a head of bushy gray hair on a thin stalk of a neck, like a dandelion. Dark coffee stains marred her misshapen teeth. A young woman was at her side, trying to support her.

"She started feeling dizzy at the end of the infusion," Malik said, referring to the Persantine drip he was using.

I asked him if he had administered aminophylline, the antidote.

"I have it here," Denis announced, holding up a syringe. "She was doing fine the whole time. Just at the end—"

"What is she feeling?" I broke in, irritated by the interruption in my schedule. "What's wrong, ma'am?"

"She doesn't speak English," Malik said. He said something to the young companion in Urdu. She repeated it loudly for the old woman, who said something in a dialect I did not understand.

"She feels weak and fatigued, and she has a headache," the young woman said.

"I am ready with the aminophylline," Denis reminded me.

"Well, what are you waiting for?" I barked. "Open your eyes, ma'am! Open . . ." I turned to her companion. "Can you tell her to open her eyes?"

When she did, bloodshot conjunctiva stared blankly at me. The young woman said something.

"What's wrong with her eyes?" I asked.

"I forgot to tell you, she is blind," Denis replied. After hooking up the syringe to her IV, he injected the aminophylline into her vein. We waited. The teetering gradually lessened. After about a minute, the old lady said she was feeling better. With Denis and her companion on either side, she stood up and was escorted to the nuclear camera to begin image acquisition. Malik tapped on the keyboard to close his report. Dreading having to see another patient, I returned to my exam room.

In the late morning I took a short break and walked up Jamaica Avenue to a nearby deli for coffee. It was one of those hole-in-the-wall joints doubling as a convenience store. The burly guy behind the counter was scraping the grill, metal on metal, waiting for an order. I ordered an omelet sandwich and poured myself a cup of coffee. The Persian cashier demanded to know why I had taken two cups. I told him that the coffee was too hot, that it was burning my hand. He gave a surly laugh. "I don't care, man, take all the cups. Throw them out. I don't care."

And so it went for the morning and early afternoon. One patient I saw was a Caribbean woman with a bewitched look who nodded off while I was examining her. I called her name a few times, getting ready to shake her, before she woke up. I asked her what was wrong, but she didn't seem to know what I was talking about. I kept pushing her, but she was infuriatingly noncommittal. ("How are you feeling?" "Not so bad now." "Are you back to normal?" "Almost." "Are you weak?" "A bit, but better.") For a moment I wondered if she'd had a seizure, but she seemed so normal afterward, not at all confused, so I let it go. I sent her to an adjoining room for an echo. A few minutes later, Eva, the sonographer, came out and told me the patient was "twitching, like." When I went in, she was lying completely still on a vinyl procedure table. She did not respond to her name or to my repeated entreaties to tell me what was wrong. What finally got her attention was when I threatened to call an ambulance.

"What for you going to call an ambulance?" she said, opening her eyes.

I told her I was afraid she was having a stroke.

"No, I get these vibrations sometimes," she explained. "Just the spirits calling me."

And was she taking medication for this condition?

"What for, medicine?" she demanded. "Just ask my son, this happen to me now and then."

"Well, please don't do it here," I said.

"You think I can control it, Doc? This been happening all my life."

"Well, if it happens again, I'm sending you to the hospital."

Though she was obviously annoyed, the spells stopped for the remainder of the procedure.

Between patients I quickly reviewed echos and nuclear scans. By then I had learned that the company providing echos to Dr. Chaudhry was run by his cousin Faisal, a chubby, mealymouthed fellow who occasionally stopped by the office to make sure I was reading his studies. The pictures were often difficult to interpret, blurry from either too little ultrasound signal or too much. But Chaudhry had instructed me not to write "technically limited" on my reports because it reflected poorly on the company.

"Amir set me up when I came here in 2006," Faisal once explained. His company was performing echos for internists and family physicians all along the South Shore and Queens. He told me companies like his were doing many things: mammograms, bone density radiographs, carotid ultrasounds, even nerve conduction studies. "Most internists are only doing EKGs in the office. If you chip in another service, they like it."

He said that doctors wanted everything done in their offices so they didn't have to worry about their patients' venturing out and being snatched up by another physician. Moreover, the imaging companies were paying them a couple of thousand dollars a month in rent. "But it isn't free money for them," Faisal said. "They have to give us patients to do echos on," which would then be reimbursed to the company by insurers. And what was in it for the patients? I asked. He replied: "Patients don't want to do a lot of driving. If you see a 7-Eleven and a Shell station, which one will you prefer?" He paused for a moment and then answered his own question. "The Shell station—because it has gas and coffee. The 7-Eleven only has coffee."

He told me that some of his competitors were outsourcing test interpretations to India, receiving reports that were generated by a machine, not a physician.

"Is that legal?" I asked, dumbfounded.

He laughed. "The market is so bad since the Russians came in. They go to school for echo; then they buy a machine and start doing tests. A doctor I know was working with one of these companies. I asked him to send me a male and a female report. They were exactly the same: same measurements, same conclusion, everything. It was all made up. Only the name was different. See, we are professionals, Dr. Jauhar. Not like those other guys."

By the time I was finished that Saturday afternoon, I had made up my mind I was going to quit. I was seeing so many patients, reading so many unnecessary tests—and Chaudhry was keeping most of the revenue anyway. Working with Chaudhry, I'd decided, was like allowing your eyes to close momentarily while driving late at night. You know it isn't a good idea. You know your judgment is impaired. But you think you can control it.

I popped my head into the treadmill room to say goodbye to Malik. He must have seen something in my expression because he put away his reports and asked me to sit down. I didn't want to talk, but I sat down anyway.

"Look, I can see you're unhappy," he said as I fidgeted like a student at the headmaster's office. "When you leave fellowship, you have this idealistic notion of the way things should be. All this running around burns you out, but it pays off in the end."

I nodded impassively.

"Amir is a businessman, you understand," Malik went on. "That's the way you have to be if you want to survive today. In my neighborhood I see electricians and plumbers. Time was, those guys couldn't afford to live in a doctor's neighborhood, but now they're making more money and doctors are making less. The status has changed."

Eva came in to tell me that my car was blocking the driveway. Always the last to arrive, I was usually the first to leave, too. I told her I'd be right out.

"Most doctors want to help people," Malik said. "But to make money for the ex-wife or the fancy house, they are starting to do stupid things. I know doctors who are doing treadmill tests on patients with emphysema who cannot exercise. Their heart rate doesn't budge, but they inject them with the isotope anyway. They know it's useless, but they don't want to lose the revenue."

"It's fraud," I said, unable to hide my disgust.

"It is," he said calmly. "Deep down they know it's wrong, which is why they are so depressed."

It occurred to me that this assessment might also apply to me. I had been practicing a sort of ethics of double effect. The double-effect principle, as I had learned at the hospital ethics committee a couple of years back, states that actions in pursuit of a good end are acceptable even if they result in a negative outcome, as long as the negative outcome is unintended and not a direct consequence of the good one.

In my case, I had been trying to meet the expenses of my family. I was putting in the extra hours so that my son could go to an independent school, not the overcrowded local one. The waste, the overtesting, were unintended, a function of circumstance. I didn't want to participate in this deception, but at the time it seemed the only way I could remain in my apartment, pay down my debt, and give my family what I thought they deserved. Of course, good intentions didn't exonerate me. Even beyond the wasted money, what about the false positives, the radiation exposure, the downstream invasive procedures? Even if I wasn't primarily responsible, even if I was just the guy following up on tests that other doctors had ordered, the consequences were the same. I used to despise the unethical behavior of doctors in private practice, but in reality I was no better than they were.

"I often wonder, Why am I doing this?" Malik said, as though reading my mind.

"Why *are* you doing this?" I asked.

"Because, like you, I have to pay my bills. But one place was so bad I had to quit. They were doing stress tests on healthy eighteen-year-olds who could run fifteen minutes on the treadmill without even breaking a sweat." He shook his head, as if to banish an uncomfortable thought. "You think New York is the worst? No, Dr. Jauhar, this kind of stuff goes on everywhere. West Coast, New Jersey—it's just the degree."

I slung my bag over my shoulder and got up. "Just try to be accommodating," he said gently, reaching out to stop me. "In the beginning, when I go to a new place, I go the extra step. Then they become dependent on you, and you can do what you want. But if you show that you don't want to do this, Chaudhry is just going to get someone else. There is only a finite amount of work, but an infinite number of doctors who are prepared to do it."

I nodded and moved to leave.

"You are very principled," he said. "But in the end, what does it get you if you go home and have a headache?" He gave a small laugh. "Anyway, make your decision and let me know. And maybe I'll see you next Saturday."

Outside, the sun was blazing, though the temperature wasn't much above freezing. I backed out of the driveway. The neighborhood was teeming with ethnic life. I drove past farmacias, halal butchers, and ninety-nine-cent taco stands. Steam rose from gutters. The whirring of the treadmill—dum-dum, dum-dum—kept reverberating through my head.

In the car I called Rajiv. If I'd expected any sympathy from him, that hope was quickly dashed.

"You don't understand!" I said as the conversation got heated. "You're his best friend. You don't have a business relationship."

"He created his empire," Rajiv snapped. "What incentive does he have to pay you more money?"

"How much do you suppose he makes on any given—"

"That is none of your concern! He is giving you an opportunity."

"Fine, but suppose he makes seven hundred dollars—"

"You are such an asshole! It's like Dad all over again!" he bellowed, referring to my father's lifelong discord with colleagues. "I want to pull my hair out when I talk to you, because you just don't get it. Or you don't want to get it."

"Calm down," I said. "I'm not saying—"

"What are you going to do if you can't find other work? They're going to foreclose on your apartment!"

"Okay, stop."

"Like Dad, you're going to screw this up and then try to fix it afterward. God, I wish I had never helped you. He is twenty percent of my cath volume! You're going to screw up my relationship with him, too!"

"It's not like that," I said weakly.

"He calls me and tells me you are late to the office. Why can't you get there on time? He is trying to run a business!"

"Listen—"

"Why don't you understand, Sandeep? You need him! He is helping you in your time of need. A year ago you were crying in my backyard. Now you're showing an attitude?"

"Stop. Just listen—"

"No, I am sick of you! You've got a good thing going, and you still don't know how to be happy. Like Dad says, you love blowing on cold milk."

"I'm not doing it on purpose."

"Dad didn't do it on purpose either," Rajiv shot back. "Look, you asked me to set this up. I leaned on my friendship. I arranged all the meetings at the hospital. Now, why the fuck do you care how much he makes! You feel he is screwing you because he gives you work. You resent him instead of appreciating the opportunity you have been given."

I kept quiet. There was a grain of truth in what Rajiv was saying. I subverted my own goals and then obsessed over the consequences. Why did I wait for a calamity before trying to change?

"He hired you only because you are my brother," Rajiv taunted me, and he was right. Chaudhry had been raised in a culture where fraternal relationships are paramount. You put up with someone's bullshit if his brother is your best friend. He was constrained by his traditions, and I had taken advantage of it.

"This is the only way you can continue to work at LIJ and still pay your bills," Rajiv said, calming down. "If you lose this, you have nothing. You will have to go into private practice full-time. You will have to do the same shit as Chaudhry and all those other doctors you despise."

"I know," I said quietly. "I don't want that."

Rajiv reminded me once again about his short time in private practice in Stony Brook, New York. "Remember that internist who called me in the middle of the night for that old lady with pneumonia? There was a rule that patients had to be seen within three hours of arriving in the ER. I told him I'd see the patient in the morning, and so he tells me, 'If you can't see her, I'll call someone else,' because he didn't want to go to the ER himself, and the message was 'Get your ass out of bed or you're going to lose my business.' I quit the next day."

I had heard this story many times. If Rajiv couldn't handle full-time private practice, there was little hope for me.

"It's just hard to do this every weekend," I said, my voice cracking. "I want to spend time with my family, too."

"This is *for* your family, Sandeep! Why don't you understand that? Maybe I'm naive, or maybe I'm a bad father for not going to every soccer game; but I really don't see the problem. You just have to do it. I mean, do you need the money? Maybe you don't need the money anymore. I don't know your situation."

"Don't be an asshole. You know I need the money."

"Well then, you have your answer, right? You don't have any options. Just remember where you were when we were playing basketball in my backyard. This is life. Nothing is free."

TEN

Moral Hazard

Passengers who insist on flying the plane are called hijackers!
—Russell B. Roth, M.D., AMA president, "A Bankrupt Law,"
American Medical News (1976), on the passage of the HMO Act

When my family arrived in the United States from New Delhi in the winter of 1977, we moved into a tiny two-bedroom house in Lexington, Kentucky, with a creaky porch and a cracked footpath that ran like an artery through the front yard. We lived simply. My sister, Suneeta, and I shared a bedroom, while Rajiv had to sleep on a cot in the dining room, next to a clanging radiator, dozing off most nights to a Cincinnati Reds ball game on his tiny transistor radio. We ate meals on a scuffed table we bought at a garage sale, which doubled as a Ping-Pong counter after Rajiv and I installed a makeshift net made of twine secured by two pencils. The house was freezing, but I don't remember our ever complaining. We took Dad at his word that President Carter had asked citizens to keep the thermostat below 65 degrees Fahrenheit to ease the energy crisis.

The one luxury we enjoyed was that on special Saturdays my parents took us to an all-you-can-eat buffet called Duff's. We'd starve ourselves until early afternoon and then pile into our white Ford Maverick compact for the drive into town. My father, dressed in polyester slacks and short sleeves, would be in the driver's seat, while my mother, in a cheap sari and overcoat, would continuously admonish him to slow down and stay clear of big trucks. By the time we made it into the crowded parking lot, it was usually three o'clock. Duff's had low wooden beams and stained-glass windows and was dark and cool, like a church. We'd wait in line, fidgety with hunger, as the savory smells drew us in. Dad's and Mom's tickets were two dollars apiece, Rajiv's and mine a dollar, and Suneeta, who was three years old, ate for free. After Dad had paid the cashier, we sprinted over to the smorgasbord of fried chicken and potatoes au gratin and trout amandine and a salad bar that stretched to the horizon, and filled our plates. We'd fill them again and again. If the chicken got cold, Dad would tell us to throw it out and get more. He wouldn't think twice about discarding an untouched piece of pecan pie if he decided he wanted a custard cream with his coffee instead. We gorged; we were wasteful; we took advantage—because it was (essentially) free. We'd eat so much that one of us would invariably get sick on the way home. When the price went up, we stopped going.

I often think of Duff's when I think about waste in health care. Someone else appears to be paying for it, so who cares how much it costs? In 1867 the *Aetna Guide to Fire Insurance* introduced the concept of moral hazard into actuarial science. The publication warned that generous insurance policies could make some people careless about preventing fires. Protected in part from the consequences of their actions, those people were more likely to engage in risky behavior, like not clearing their yards of brush or leaving their houses without adequate ventilation. The guide made a revolutionary and counterintuitive point: insurance in some cases can increase risk.

Moral hazard undoubtedly plays a role in health care, too. When people complain that their rising insurance premiums are funding others' irresponsible behavior, they are complaining about moral hazard. When patients with low-deductibility insurance go to the emergency room for a hangnail, they are succumbing to moral hazard. When a nurse in the ICU criticizes a family for refusing to authorize a DNR order ("They would never do this if they had to pay for it"), she is talking about moral hazard. The moral hazard hypothesis was put to the test in the 1970s with the RAND Health Insurance Experiment. For a decade it followed eight thousand people who had been randomly assigned to one of five types of health insurance plan: an HMO-style group cooperative or a traditional plan that covered 100 percent, 95 percent, 50 percent, or 25 percent of costs. Predictably, the study found that medical spending was highest when 100 percent of costs were covered. If health care is perceived as free, patients will demand more of it.

Moral hazard is at play on the provider side, too. Chest pains? Why not order a stress test when the nuclear camera is in the next room. Palpitations? Get a Holter monitor—and throw in an echocardiogram for good measure. It is too easy to prescribe tests when you know an insurance company will pay for them. "Supply may induce its own demand [when] a third party practically guarantees reimbursement," wrote the authors of the Dartmouth Atlas Project, and there are strong data to support this assertion. For example, the number of freestanding diagnostic imaging centers owned by doctors or private investors has more than doubled during the past decade. A doctor who owns a nuclear scanner is seven times as likely as other doctors to call for a scan. The growth in the volume of imaging services has far outstripped the growth of all other physician services. In 2006, Americans were exposed to seven times the amount of radiation than they had been in 1987, primarily because of CT scans, which now number more than seventy million per year.

Of course, many forces, including new and expensive technology, the aging of the population, and the rise of chronic diseases, are behind increasing imaging costs. But moral hazard undoubtedly plays a role. Managed care, with its reliance on high deductibles and capitation, in which physicians are paid a set amount per assigned patient, whether or not that patient seeks care, came of age with the idea of controlling moral hazard. In the 1970s many insurers adopted co-payments to increase the price of medical care to consumers in an effort to reduce inefficient spending. In the 1980s and 1990s, economists promoted fixed payments and utilization review, in which payers approve or deny requests for medical services, to further reduce moral hazard. The managed care system that we know today is largely a product of this theory. And though it worked for a while—health expenditures slowed significantly in the 1980s and 1990s, the heyday of managed care—patient and physician revulsion against third-party interference in medical decision-making eventually forced many insurers to back away from these unpopular cost-cutting strategies. Health care spending has accelerated once again over the past decade.

After the blowup with Rajiv, I committed myself to changing my stand-offish ways. Rajiv had been urging me for some time to meet socially with his physician friends in a relaxed atmosphere away from the hospital, and so there I was a few weeks later at a doctors' party in Manhasset, a tony suburb on the North Shore of Long Island. The host, a Sikh internist with a bright red turban, greeted me warmly when I arrived. "Rajiv is my best friend," he said, putting his arm around me and showing me to the foyer where shoes were stowed. "We have heard so much about you."

I found Rajiv in the dining room playing an Indian card game called teen patti. He was cracking jokes, holding court, acting every bit like the Indian mensch he was reputed to be. When he saw me, he bounded over, obviously tipsy. "I'm glad you came," he said, giving me a hug. He handed me an empty tumbler. "My bro is here," he cried to the host. "Break out the good shit!"

Rajiv went back to his card game while I stood awkwardly in the middle of the room. Turning to the oncologist sitting next to him, he said, "All right, asshole, now place a real bet. It isn't even one co-pay." When the doctor quickly folded, Rajiv said, "Don't worry, the next bone marrow biopsy is on me."

Someone piped in: "The next anemia consult is on me."

I went to the kitchen and poured myself a Scotch. Out in the living room, a group of mostly male doctors were relaxing on couches and fold-out chairs, drinking Black Label and chatting comfortably. I sat down next to a lanky Gujarati doctor in private practice whom I'd met several times on the wards at LIJ. "Haven't seen you in a while," I said, trying to sound pleasant and familiar. He nodded politely and turned his attention back to the conversation.

"I tell you, medicine has been taken out of our hands and put into the hands of uneducated people," a Punjabi internist perched at the edge of the sofa was saying. Apparently he had sold his practice about a year prior and was now working part-time at a hospital in Brooklyn. He recalled some of the annoyances when he was practicing full-time. "Insurance companies would put restrictions on almost every medication. I'd get a call: 'Drug not covered. Write a different prescription or get pre-authorization.' If I ordered an MRI, I'd have to explain to a clerk why I wanted to do the test. It was a big, big headache."

When he decided to work for a hospital, he figured there would be more freedom to practice his specialty. "But managed care is like a magnet attached to you. They say you didn't take authorization for this test. I tell the girl, 'Why should I take authorization from you? You're not a doctor. You just read about this in some book.'"

"It is getting so bad," someone responded. "They want us to practice perfect medicine, but they put up barriers at every inch."

"I have to spend hours on the phone getting precertification," a Jewish family doctor said. "I order a drug and the patient calls me up and says the insurance company won't approve it, and somehow it is my responsibility to fight the company for them. Part of me wants to say, 'I ordered the drug; I did the right thing. Now fight your own battles.'"

"People think we are greedy," Dr. Oni, the Nigerian internist with "consultitis," declared. "But look at these insurance companies. For some of them it is written into the medical director's contract to deny every fourth admission." (I had heard a similar charge from a billing clerk at my hospital.)

"Thirty percent of my admissions are being denied," the Punjabi internist replied. "There is a forty-five-day limit on the appeal. If you don't bill in time, you lose everything. You're discussing this with some guy on the phone, and you think, You're sitting there, I'm sitting here. How do you know anything about this patient?"

"It is all about the money," Oni asserted. "Look at these capitated insurance programs. They say they will pay fifteen dollars a year per patient. Now, can you see a patient for fifteen dollars? Even if you see her once a year, is that enough?"

"Why did you sign the contract?" someone demanded.

"Because doctors are not united," Oni replied to murmurs of agreement. "If you say no, you know Dr. B or Dr. C will say yes. They will get the contract and the patients. It is still money, even if it is not a lot.

"An internist like me," he went on. "Let's say you want a certain salary to meet your family's expenses. That means you have to double it to pay your overhead. I used to have a nurse. That's one hundred thousand dollars a year. A physician's assistant is ninety thousand. A nurse practitioner is one hundred and ten thousand. Who can afford it? You have to bring in half a million just to achieve your salary goal. I used to see fifteen patients a day. Now reimbursement is so low I have to see at least thirty. If I stay in the room more than ten minutes, my assistant will call me and tell me to hurry up."

He said he was doing a plethora of tests—eye exams, audiometry, pulmonary function tests, even Holter monitoring—to generate revenue in the office. "You ask yourself, which doctor would you want to go to? One who does every test, never mind that they are normal"—he laughed bitterly—"or one who doesn't do such a thorough job? A lot of this is also being driven by patients asking for tests."

I'd heard a similar assessment from Chaudhry. Quietly listening, I nursed my drink.

The Punjabi internist said that he used to work with a pulmonologist. "To bill for lung spirometry, he would have the patient quickly blow into a tube. He didn't even look at the results. We did stress tests, too. We knew who was going to be normal. We avoided the high-risk cases, the asthmatics and the hypertensives." He laughed. "Those we would send to a cardiologist."

A gastroenterologist with waxy brown hair said: "If a doctor doesn't do excess testing, forget it, he isn't going to be able to live. This is the only profession in the world where you can provide a service and not know if you are going to be paid for it."

Oni said he had received payments from a mobile echo company for referring patients for cardiac ultrasounds. Though he no longer participated in these contracts, he was open about the fees—about $100 per patient, paid in cash—and he saw nothing wrong with it. "As internists, we don't do procedures, so we have to figure out another way to make money. But it isn't hard once you figure out how to do it."

"We don't clock the number of minutes when we talk with our patients," someone said. "We don't hang up the phone as lawyers may do if they are not going to get paid. No, we listen to patients and answer their questions, however long it takes."

The family doctor suggested that patients call a toll number if they wanted to speak to their physicians. "Sure, I'll talk to you," he said. "Just call this 888 number. I'll talk to you as long as you want. I'll even talk dirty to you." People laughed. "My lawyer always tells me, 'If I'm thinking about your case, even while I'm taking a leak, you're getting charged three hundred and fifty dollars an hour.'"

Oni said, "I have a cousin who is an ob-gyn. He is paying one hundred and fifty thousand dollars a year for malpractice insurance. As an obstetrician, you have to earn five hundred thousand dollars just to make ends meet. That is why people don't want to do it anymore."

"I did obstetrics," someone replied. "They used to pay fifty-five hundred dollars for fourteen office visits plus a delivery when you stay up all night. Now they pay twenty-four hundred. You think that's reasonable? Your wife delivered. Is that enough money to make it worthwhile?" He shook his head, disgusted. "The problem is, they cut the money, they took away the autonomy, but they didn't take away any of the responsibility."

"It is getting tougher and tougher," the only female doctor in the room declared. "Everyone is looking for procedures. I feel sorry for the patients. We're sending them here and there, for this test and that. Sometimes I tell them, 'Go home. You've had every test. There is nothing more for me to do.' I said to my husband, in a few years, when the mortgage is paid off, I want to do something else. This is not the concept of medicine I had when I started."

Back in the kitchen, I poured myself another drink. Rajiv came over. Now drunk, he slapped me hard on the back. "You should talk to Dr. Shah," he said. "Give him your card, your cell phone, your beeper. Tell him to call you anytime."

I nodded and looked away.

"I still can't believe you came," Rajiv said. "Are you having a good time?"

———

A few months later, in the midst of the global financial crisis of 2008, I went to Parents' Night at Mohan's preschool on the Upper West Side. The party had a Polynesian theme, and the gymnasium was replete with luau decorations and hula dancers. At the tiki bar I ran into an old friend, Stephen, who had dropped out of medical school at Cornell twenty years earlier to pursue investment banking. Whenever we meet, Stephen always seems to find a way to congratulate me on what he considers my professional calling. He often wonders whether he should have stuck with medicine. Like many expatriates, he has idealistic notions of the world he left.

That night we talked about the tumult on Wall Street. Like many of

his colleagues, he was worried about the future. He did not foresee continuing rewards for what he had been trained to do.

"It's a good time to be a doctor," Stephen declared. "I'd love a job
where I didn't have to constantly think about money."

I must have rolled my eyes. Feeling sorry for him, I assured him that
his business would bounce back.

He shrugged. "I'm okay right now. I mean, my wife and I were able
to put away some money—about ten million dollars—so I'm secure. But
I'd like to make more."

Ten million? And I was worried about making next month's nursery
school payment.

Though I didn't bother to disillusion Stephen, most doctors today,
whether in academic or private practice, have to constantly think about
money, too. In 2009, Dr. Pamela Hartzband and her husband, Dr. Je-
rome Groopman, physicians at Beth Israel Deaconess Medical Center
in Boston, wrote in *The New England Journal of Medicine* that "price
tags are being applied to every aspect of a doctor's day, creating an acute
awareness of costs and reimbursement." They added: "Today's medical
students are being inducted into a culture in which their profession is
seen increasingly in financial terms."

The rising commercialism has obvious consequences for the public:
ballooning costs, harm to patients, and fraying of the traditional doctor-
patient bond. What is not so obvious to most people is the harmful effects
on doctors themselves. We were trained to think like caregivers, not busi-
nesspeople. The constant intrusion of the marketplace has created serious and deepening anxiety in our profession.

Not long ago, a cardiology fellow who had been interviewing for jobs
came to my office, clearly disillusioned. "I was naive," he said. "I'd never
thought of medicine as a business. I thought we were in it to take care of
patients. But I guess it is."

I asked him how he felt about going into private practice. "I won't
have much time to think about it," he replied. "I'll be too busy vomiting
for the first six months."

Certainly, there has always been a profit motive in medicine, but financial considerations have never been as prominent as they are today,
in part because so many hospitals and doctors, especially in large metropolitan areas, are in financial trouble. Even as payments by insurers are

decreasing inexorably to control health costs, office expenses are increasing, and the economy is in recession. More and more doctors are trying to sell their practices or are negotiating with hospitals for jobs, equipment, or financial aid. At academic medical centers, uncompensated care is growing as patients suffering from the economic downturn lose health insurance. Admissions and elective procedures—big moneymakers— are declining. Hospitals are cutting administrative costs, staff, and services in an effort to remain profitable.

Of course, the blame for this commercialization doesn't lie exclusively with doctors and hospitals. Politicians, insurers, drug companies, and even patients bear some responsibility, too. We are all in a tragic cycle of action and reaction, in which each party pursues its own ends without sight of the big picture, making the system more and more diseased. Self-interest doesn't always work for the greater good. On the ramp to the expressway, you need lights to modulate the flow of traffic. Otherwise you get a jam.

Despite this, a part of me still wants to see doctors master the business side of our profession. When I hear about executives at health companies getting tens of millions of dollars in bonuses, the blatant profiteering sickens me. As a member of the guild, I want to see doctors exert more control over our financial house.

And yet the consequences of this commercial consciousness are troubling. Among my colleagues I see an emotional emptiness created by the relentless consideration of money. Most of us went into medicine for intellectual stimulation or the desire to develop relationships with patients, not to maximize income. There is a palpable sense of grieving. The job for many has become just that—a job.

Something fundamental is lost when physicians start thinking of medicine as a business. In their essay, Hartzband and Groopman talk about the erosion of collegiality, cooperation, and teamwork when a marketplace environment takes hold in the hospital. "The balance has tipped toward market exchanges at the expense of medicine's communal or social dimension," they write.

The result, as I witnessed at the Manhasset party, is exhaustion, depersonalization, and burnout. Approximately a third of physicians surveyed admit to signs of burnout. Burnout is associated with excessive workload, difficulty balancing one's personal and professional lives, and loss of work control, autonomy, and meaning. It has been described as "an erosion of the soul caused by a deterioration of one's values, dignity, spirit and will." The practice of medicine today almost seems to promote burnout. Doctors are working harder and harder, and many continue to demand perfection of themselves. We defer gratification, sometimes for many years. We no longer feel in charge of our professional destiny. A physician recently wrote online: "The reason we are feeling 'burnout' is that there does not seem to be any hope for things to get better." Another said, speaking for many in private practice who stand to lose the most from policy proposals to restrict fee-for-service and encourage greater use of nurse practitioners and physician's assistants to do what was formerly doctors' work, "We look forward to a future of a fully implemented Obamacare where physicians are but meaningless pawns in the hands of those who are pushing this absurd social experiment." Such irrational anger, the almost operatic self-pity, has become commonplace. I encountered it countless times those first few years at LIJ. Colleagues would complain: We are not being allowed to work in a market economy. We are not being allowed to charge what the market will bear, or for what we should be able to charge on the basis of our expenses and our education, thanks to the "price-fixing" that starts with Medicare and trickles down to other insurers. And yet there was almost never a sense that we were to blame, too. That we had abandoned our course. That many doctors had abused the public trust and taken advantage of the system. Doctors never seem to acknowledge that the widespread burnout in our profession is in part due to the behavior of doctors themselves.

ELEVEN

Devotion

What we call fate does not come into us from the outside, but emerges from us.   —Rainer Maria Rilke, *Letters to a Young Poet*, 1929

It was getting harder and harder to get started with the mundane tasks of the day. I was doing what was generally expected of me—the moonlighting, my regular job at LIJ, and, beyond that, taking Mohan to the park or Sonia out for dinner on weekends when I wasn't on call—but I was getting accustomed to thinking that a three-quarters effort would almost always be enough. A kind of sluggishness had taken hold: a vague sort of queasiness, a hint of something that I was supposed to want but that was somehow beyond my reach, and a fear that I was not going to be able to let go of this feeling, that it was going to stay with me for some time. Sometimes I wanted to cry, but I almost never did. Even when tears did flow—for instance, at the conclusion of a marital spat ("Why are you so checked out, Sandeep?") or after an unexpectedly kind comment from a friend or colleague—the relief was transient, and the heaviness always returned. This was a different kind of fear from what I had experienced in my youth, not so much of what the future was going to bring but that it had already arrived.

I wasn't alone, of course; there is an enormous reservoir of subterranean depression in middle age. A recent study of two million adults in eighty countries found that middle age is the time in our lives when we are most likely to be unhappy. Regardless of wealth, gender, or social, marital, or filial status, the pattern is largely the same: happiness peaks in our twenties, dips in our forties, and rises again when we are older. Though one in five people will experience depression at some point in life, the frequency is highest among middle-aged adults. Men in their forties and fifties have the highest suicide rate, three times the national average. Among professionals, physicians have the highest suicide rate. One American doctor kills himself or herself every day.

————

Sonia had been practicing yoga for many years. Growing up in the Indian enclave of Edison, New Jersey, she had spent considerable time in the company of gurus who came to her home every week to engage in prayer and satsangs (spiritual dialectics) with her father. Some in her extended family had followed the teachings of several famous yogis, including one I remembered from newscasts in the early 1980s.

"Wasn't he the guy with the Rolls-Royces?"

"Yes, well, he did some bad things," Sonia replied. "But they say he was a genius."

"Wasn't he screwing young women?"

"I don't know. But he was enlightened!"

After we got married, Sonia discovered a deep-breathing exercise called Sudarshan Kriya that was touted to alleviate stress and anxiety. The few times she made me try it ("Don't people in midlife crises investigate new religions?"), I did feel more relaxed (probably acute respiratory alkalosis caused by rapid ventilation, I hypothesized). I'd read about the benefits of yoga: stress reduction, beneficial changes in blood chemistry, better sleep patterns, decreased resting heart rate, etc. So in late November 2007, when the guru who had popularized kriya visited Sonia's parents' home in Edison, I went to meet him. I was looking for something that would lessen the weight in my chest, and even though I'd never had a strong religious faith, I was still hoping to reap some benefits from Guruji's purported wisdom.

My father-in-law picked me up at the train station in his black Mercedes. It was an overcast day, and the trees along the road were leafless and gray. I felt the strange disquietude that autumn always seems to bring, only that year it was more intense than usual. We passed by doctors' offices, physical therapy suites, and MRI centers—the drab medical-industrial complex of the Garden State in its concrete glory. Stopping at a traffic light, my father-in-law broke the silence. "The water is the same, whether it splashes you in winter or summer," he said, staring ahead. "It is your sensation that changes."

I looked over at him and nodded politely. I knew he was trying to help me, even if I didn't know what he was talking about.

"We have control over our responses," he said. "We can choose to be happy or not."

I nodded again, feigning understanding. Though he was a successful doctor, my father-in-law more than anything was an aging mystic.

"You should think that everything is going to change for the better," he went on encouragingly. "Think: I have never been born; I will never die. This embodiment is around my eternal bliss. Try to relate to that bliss." He touched his chest. "It is yours. You just need to tap into it."

A Sanskrit devotional was playing on the stereo. He recited a verse from it, which he translated: "'You have bred an explosion of joy in my heart, so that I am floating on a breeze'—like you float on the ocean when you are surfing," he added, interrupting himself. "'And I am feeling a breath of fresh air flowing all over me.'" He turned to me, looking mesmerized. "It is a beautiful ghazal about prana. Do you know what prana is?"

"Is it energy?"

"No, it is breath; it is life. When someone dies, we say, 'Prana khatam,' meaning 'He took his last breath.' Guruji says you can direct the prana. Like when we prayed that you and Sonia would have children."

The light turned green. The car jerked forward. I went back to staring out the window.

"One day I have to sit down and explain to you the meaning of all these things," he said. (He had been promising this for some time.) "I'm sure the mind has healing powers. I see it all the time in the hospital. People who are depressed or angry don't do as well."

I nodded but didn't say anything. Nothing would have made me happier at that moment than to feel different.

"Believe in the power of prayer," he went on. "There is a lot of evidence that prayer by or for you promotes healing." I wasn't so sure. I'd seen the pattern many times. Sonia's father would pray for someone who was sick, and she would get better, and he'd attribute the recovery to prayer, but that person was probably at the tail end of her viral illness anyway.

"The key is to be happy," he declared as we pulled onto his street. "Happy every single moment of your life. Be happy, not angry. It makes me sad to see you this way."

The house was a whitewashed colonial sitting on thirty acres at the end of a long tree-lined gravel drive. Sonia met us at the back entrance, looking relaxed in jeans and a sweater, obviously pleased that I had made the trip. We went inside, where shoes had been stowed in a foyer alongside statues of Hindu deities. A poster-size picture of Guruji hung over the doorway leading into the living room. I saw him sitting on the rug. He had long black hair intermingled with thick gray strands and a long, flowing beard. He was wearing an orange vest that revealed hairy armpits. People, hands clasped, were kneeling before him, vying for his attention. A young man in an argyle sweater was curled up at the entryway, looking crazed. "I feel so incredibly close to him," I heard him say. "He feels like a dear, dear friend."

The house was overrun with Guruji's devotees: wealthy Indians, middle-class Indians, crunchy-granola whites. In the kitchen a group of his disciples were assembled at a table, participating in a kind of dialectic. The leader, a young woman with a blond ponytail, was explaining that kriya meditation had to be practiced regularly. "You must do it for at least forty consecutive days," she said with spurious precision. "That is how long it takes to integrate into your system. Anything less than forty days, you will have to start all over again. If you do it for thirty-seven days and then skip a day, you will have to start from day one."

Someone asked about how to conquer unhappiness. The key, the young woman replied, was to dispense with desire. "Expectations kill the joy," she declared. I had heard this axiom many times, but it had never made much sense to me. Doesn't such a strategy conquer happiness, too? Isn't desire just an appetite for joy?

People seemed to know the house belonged to a doctor because the discussion quickly turned to health and disease. A woman outfitted in a bright sari and sparkling jewelry said she had recently been diagnosed with diabetes, with a blood sugar level of 400, dangerously high. "Doctors said that if I had waited a couple of days, I would have gone into a coma," she said, seemingly directing her comments at me. Now her blood sugar was controlled with "a single pill only," a situation that she attributed to the power of Guruji. "It was a miracle," she said. "How can anyone deny this was a miracle?"

I couldn't help thinking that a $10 co-pay was the best deal on a miracle she was ever going to get.

She said that she had once seen Guruji in her bedroom in the middle of the night. "I woke my husband and told him there was somebody in the house," she recalled. "I was scared, but I knew it was Guruji; I knew he had come." About a half hour later, she said, Guruji called her from India and asked if she had called him. Terrified, she hung up the phone, but she dialed him the next day. "I asked, 'Guruji, were you in my house last night?' and he said yes." She looked around the table. "Now, you tell me that is not a miracle."

I stared at her impassively.

"I kept saying, 'I can't believe this,'" her husband said. It was evidence, to him, of "superpower."

Another person said that he had recently been on a plane set to fly to Sedona, Arizona, but that he did not want to go. A few minutes before takeoff, with 150 passengers on board, the flight got canceled. He was sure this had some special meaning.

"Perhaps it was a coincidence," I blurted out before Sonia pinched me. People always seemed to want to attribute a grand design to random events. It required a constant recalibration of one's thinking that I found disingenuous and dangerous. "What about the folks who wanted to go to Sedona?" I said.

"They didn't want to go either," the man replied pleasantly. "They just didn't know it."

A pudgy middle-aged man standing next to me whispered, "Hi, I'm like you. I also hear these stories and the other side of my mind wonders, Is it real? Is this the only explanation? So you must be thinking the same thing."

I nodded politely.

"Guruji protects all his devotees," the man said.

"Why doesn't he protect everyone?" I asked.

"Because we are in his inner circle," he replied. Then he quickly added, "You must have faith, Doctor. It all depends on faith."

As a boy I'd had faith. I'd believed there were people who possessed special knowledge that I could not access. When I was in trouble, I prayed. But this all had changed. I no longer believed in prayer. I no longer trusted there was a greater source of truth than the thoughts in my own head. I was now apt to ignore the pronouncements of those in authority. Still, I missed that time when I thought others knew more than I about how to live my life. As much as the need for their approval had once unnerved me, my lack of faith was just as unsettling.

Since Sonia's family was playing host, I was accorded a coveted seat next to Guruji in the living room. He was delivering a mini satsang, saying things like "War cannot exist without peace" and making other such pithy pronouncements. Every once in a while he answered his cell phone or checked it for text messages. Sitting next to me on the floor was a young woman with ash blond hair and purple toenails, wearing yellow sweat pants and a Rutgers sweatshirt. She would cry out every once in a while with the annoying shriek of a true believer.

"This body is the temple of the Lord," Guruji declared to murmurs of assent. "Our purpose is to use this body for good. Not by going to middle schools and high schools talking religion, but rather spirituality. Spirituality and religion are very different. Spirituality unites; religion divides." He paused for a moment. "Write that down," he commanded an assistant.

After Guruji had finished his sermon, we were instructed to prostrate ourselves before him and touch his feet. After doing so, I was handed a metal plate sprinkled with rose petals and red powder. I moved it in a circular fashion in front of him and passed it along. A few of his disciples stared at me, seemingly jealous of my proximity.

Guruji asked us to write down some things we wished for but did not have. On a piece of paper I scribbled: "spontaneity and joy of childhood; peace and harmony in my marriage; self-confidence and centeredness." Then he asked us what we wanted from the practice of kriya. I wrote, "I hope to get a means to put myself in a confident frame of mind—"

Before I could finish writing, Guruji suddenly spoke up. "What do you say now? Talk!" he commanded.

An elderly woman in a drab yellow and purple sari made an appeal on behalf of her sick mother. "When she takes her medicine, she gets tight in the shoulders and shivers," she said.

"How old is your mother?" Guruji asked gruffly.

"Ninety-four," the woman replied.

There was silence, as Guruji appeared to collect his thoughts. "It will go away in due time," he said. People began to laugh.

"But it is only you, Guruji," the woman persisted, seemingly oblivious of the morbid joke. "Your powers are keeping her healthy."

"She is ninety-four!" he cried. "You worry too much about your mother."

Sonia's father stood up. He was now wearing beige kurta pajamas and had a streak of red powder on his forehead. "Guruji, this is my son-in-law, Sandeep." All eyes turned to me. "I mentioned him to you before. He is a doctor and a writer. He writes for *The New York Times.*"

I nodded respectfully. My father-in-law's remarks were a bit surprising to me because he had long attributed my problems to identity confusion. "You have to decide what you want to be," he'd said to me many times. "Doctor, writer, father—you have to make some choices."

But now, before the group, he evinced only caring and pride. "He is a physicist and a scholar, too," my father-in-law continued. "But his mind is restless. I would request you to speak with him."

Guruji regarded me with intense curiosity. No one spoke. "So what is the problem?" he said.

A warm wave washed over me, and my mind started to race: *I don't know. On the surface things seem all right, yet I feel unsettled. I keep thinking there is something to worry about, but I can't remember what it is. I am waking up with a fear that things are going to fall apart. I am dreading it, but it isn't happening, so I keep waiting, almost wishing it would happen and be over with.*

Of course, I didn't say any of this. I just stared at him. "I don't know," I replied.

Guruji smiled sympathetically. "If you have a problem, you must go to the right person," he said, as though reciting a line he had uttered many times. "A problem with your house, you go to the builder; a problem with e-mail, the engineer. And if you have a problem of spirit, you must take the advice of a guru."

The woman next to me let out another piercing shriek.

"Disease occurs when one of the five elements of the body is off," Guruji went on. "If a patient has loose motions, what does the doctor give? Saline through an IV. He treats dehydration with water. When it is cold, he gives you a blanket. For lack of soil in the body, you eat. When you are suffocating, he administers oxygen."

He stopped, waiting for a response, but no one said anything.

"The fifth element is peace of mind," he continued. "And what does the doctor do? He gives shock therapy. He treats stress with more stress!"

People murmured appreciatively. The woman beside me was now rocking back and forth and moaning.

"Yogis have a different way," Guruji continued. "Your mind is the most wonderful computer. Man has made powerful computers, but nothing compares with the brain, which is natural. Scientists have allowed us to send e-mails, but before there were computers, the old yogis were sending e-mails back and forth only through their minds."

I glanced at Guruji's buzzing cell phone and nodded.

"My mission is to convey to the world the ancient scientific wisdom of the yogis," Guruji went on. "The yogis knew that elements could be transformed into others just by changing the number of electrons. You go from four to six electrons, and you can change iron into gold! The yogis have known this for thousands of years."

He was talking like one of those crackpots who attended the Berkeley physics colloquiums on Wednesday afternoons, spewing theories about things they did not understand. And yet even though I was skeptical and knew his reasoning was faulty, I needed help. I still wanted to hear what he had to tell me.

"The universe is three things: water, matter, and vapor. And these things when you get to a small enough scale all look the same. What is the smallest unit of matter?" he demanded. I hesitated. "Atoms," he said. "And what is the makeup of the atom?" My mind was blank. "The universe itself," he answered. "The whole universe is in the tiny atom. The power is all there." He touched his forehead. "We just need to tap into it."

People sounded exclamations of agreement.

"There is no question that you will find happiness," Guruji said, quieting the group. "Just utter this mantra." He whispered a few words. "If you say this several times a day, you will enter my magnetic field. The physicists have explained that a big magnet can make smaller magnets. Magnets are everywhere: earth, stars, moons, even atoms. If you do this, you will become a magnet, too."

I nodded, feeling exhausted. Guruji stood up and announced that he was going upstairs to rest. The crowd parted to let him through.

The woman next to me remained on the floor, quietly sobbing. Tissues were wadded up into a ball on the rug. She was unable to speak. Someone said there was a remedy and dashed off to get it. He returned promptly, holding a banana.

Getting ready to leave Edison that night, I still felt the same sense of foreboding. My chest was still tight, a reminder that things weren't right. Overall, the whole experience seemed to have been a wash. In the expansive foyer, as people were milling around in small groups, chatting, one of Guruji's disciples came up to me. He was a stocky man in his fifties with a scruffy beard and a short graying ponytail, wearing a khadi jacket, leather sandals, and blue jeans that looked as if they needed washing. "Once you know and accept you are going to die," he told me with a pleasant glint in his eye, "the future will not haunt you." It was a line out of one of Guruji's pamphlets, and he said it had given him succor in difficult times. I turned the dictum around in my head. More than anything else I'd heard that evening, the words had a ring of truth. I thanked him for the advice. Then I went to find Sonia to say goodbye. Shortly afterward I got into my father-in-law's Mercedes for the ride back to the train station.

TWELVE

Denial

Private practice today is like surfing. If you don't stay on top of it, you
could go under real quick. —Comment overheard in doctors' lounge

Sonia had gone to a board review course in Cleveland. When she returned, on a staid, languid Sunday afternoon, Mohan and I went to pick
her up at the airport.

In the Lincoln Tunnel on the way there, Mohan, strapped into the
child seat in the back of the car, complained, "We're going so long,
Dadda. I can't see the clouds or the trees or the sky."

I said it was because we were stuck in a tunnel.

"What? We're stuck?"

"No, we're not *stuck*," I said quickly. "We're just going very slow." I
discerned some relief in his face.

"You know what this is called?" I said.

"Lincoln Tunnel."

"What does the Lincoln Tunnel mean?"

"It goes underwater, under the Hudson River."

"That's right!" I smiled proudly, amazed that in three and a half short
years my son had already developed into a thinking person.

When we met Sonia at the curb, she cried, "Mohan, I missed you so
much, my darling. Did you miss me?"

"Guess what?" he said. "A big blue rocket goes up really fast."

Sonia smiled. "Does he seem bigger to you? I can see he's grown,
he's more verbal."

She'd been away only a few days, but she was probably right. I said, "Mohan, Mama is going back to being a doctor soon. She is going to start working."

He didn't respond.

"Mohan, do you want to be a doctor?" I asked.

"No, a nurse."

"Not a doctor?" Sonia said.

"No, I like nurses. They take care of people."

————

I had been taking most of Chaudhry's doc-of-the-day calls. Over a twenty-four-hour period, several times a month, I admitted cardiac patients from the ER who did not already have cardiologists. However, insurance companies were denying the necessity of (and therefore payments for) about 30 percent of these admissions, meaning a lot of lost revenue for Chaudhry's practice. Chaudhry had been grousing that I wasn't bringing in enough money to cover the salary he was paying me, so I became more aggressive about appealing the rejections, which until then I had been ignoring.

"Yes, this is the CareAllies medical director."

"This is Dr. Jauhar. I called a couple of times yesterday. I know you're aware of it; but you didn't call me back, and this is the second time I'm calling today."

"I apologize for that. What can I do for you, Dr. Jauhar?"

"It is clearly stated in the appeals document that I've read and shown to people in my department that you are supposed to take my phone calls."

"Dr. Jauhar, I'm . . . there's nothing I can say. I am sorry we didn't get back to you in a more timely manner."

"As you probably know from my messages, I want to discuss the denial on James Castle."

"I am not able to approve this admission, Doctor. As our nurse informed you yesterday, this chest pain workup did not have to be done in the hospital. I understand you may disagree with this judgment, and you do have the option of an appeal. The best thing is to have your hospital send us a copy of the chart."

"To whom?"

"To CareAllies, along with the denial."

"I don't understand. This was a fifty-four-year-old smoker who was having palpitations and chest pain. Why do you feel he didn't need to be admitted to the hospital?"

"Doctor, I am not in any way questioning the services that you rendered in an extremely timely manner. But those services could have been done under an observation level of care."

"But we don't have an observation unit at my hospital!"

"I am sorry, Doctor, but that does not oblige us to pay for a level of care that was not warranted."

Whatever the case, it meant Chaudhry and I weren't getting paid. I sent in the required paperwork, filled out the appropriate appeal forms, and followed up to make sure they were received. But we never did get reimbursed for that admission.

When I checked with Liam, a billing clerk in my department, he told me that payment denials by managed care companies had become routine. "You have to take out the shovel and dig hard to get paid what's rightfully yours," he said. "By the time I'm done digging, we probably get paid about eighty percent of the time. But it isn't easy. They have all sorts of excuses: 'didn't get billed right,' 'didn't get it on time.' Come on, 'didn't get it on time'? I have three confirmations, and you're going to tell me you didn't get it on time? Please. Sometimes they won't release the funds; then you ask them and they say, 'Oh, yeah, now I see. Don't know why that wasn't paid. I'll release the funds.' My boss hears me saying on the phone, 'How's the baby, Alice?' and there's a reason for that. You have to get the insurance company on your side. I can't say, 'Hey, I want to get paid.' I have to say, 'How are you?' That works better than anything else."

As the months wore on, Chaudhry was beginning to sound irritated whenever we spoke. "I thought I was making money on you," he said on the phone one morning. "But when Jean, the biller, sent me this report, I had no choice but to talk to you and say, 'Sandeep, this is ridiculous.'"

I closed the door to my office so the conversation would not carry into the hallway. "I can give you some money back," I said quietly, even though I knew it had already been spent. "I don't want to keep your money if it isn't being earned."

"Any investor will invest if the revenue is coming in," Chaudhry said, ignoring the offer. "The problem is when the revenue is not coming. You know how much I am now getting for stress tests after expenses, Sandeep? Two hundred dollars. You know how much Oxford is paying me for a new consult? Ninety-eight dollars, and only twenty-two for a follow-up! I am taking home just enough money to pay my bills."

I was dubious, but I kept quiet. I needed to keep the moonlighting going for as long as possible, and I was afraid of saying something that could make Chaudhry terminate the deal. Nonetheless, I didn't know how much longer I could go on denying the unseemly reality of it all.

"The problem, Sandeep, is that your hospital patients are not following up in my office for tests," he said. I told him that I had been handing out his business card and offering the patients timely appointments to see me on Saturdays when I came to the office. I did not understand why they weren't coming.

"Hospital patients have their own doctors," Chaudhry explained in the pedantic tone he had increasingly been using with me. "When they go back to their internists and ask for a referral for Chaudhry or Jauhar, the internist will say, 'Why are you going there? Go to this other cardiologist. I know him.' So the chance of those patients coming to us is maybe five or ten percent. What you are doing is not wrong. This is just the dynamic of private practice."

In order to capture more of my doc-of-the-day admissions, Chaudhry told me that in addition to passing out his card, he wanted me to call Samantha, his office manager, with every patient's demographic information, as well as to fax her the insurance information. Though I was offended at having to do such scut work, I said I would.

"If you want to increase your revenue, Sandeep, you have to get into the practice," he urged. "We must figure out why more doctors are not sending us patients. What is the reason?" He mentioned that even Dr. Oni, the Nigerian internist, had stopped referring patients to the office.

Oni had been one of Chaudhry's most loyal referral sources, supporting him from the time Chaudhry opened his practice in 2002. When I started taking ER calls, Chaudhry had instructed me to refer my patients to Oni for general medicine consults to give him some extra business. I had done this for a while, but in recent months I'd stopped.

"If you send one or two extra patients to Oni, it will help us in the long run," Chaudhry lectured. "See, this is called connection. At the end of the day everybody should be happy. I'm not saying send every single patient to Oni—you don't want people to think it is automatic— but keep him in the loop. How did I get a connection with Dr. Mazer? If I have a GI issue, I use him. If he has a cardiac issue, he uses me. This is called channeling."

Chaudhry proposed a new plan. He wanted me to start seeing patients at various internists' offices where he was paying rent (essentially a fee to sit on their premises and see their patients), referring those patients back to his main office if they needed cardiac procedures. "Right now I am giving you a piece of my pie, but we have to make the pie bigger if we want this to work."

I told him I would try.

"You will be a great asset to me if you can go to Ozone Park," he said; it was about an hour's drive from my apartment. "I also have a connection in the Bronx. Just give me a few months the way I am explaining, and you will see a huge difference in your revenue."

"What about stress tests and echos?" I asked. By now I had learned the real money was in testing.

"I can give you some studies," he said. "But then you have to come to the office to read them. The problem, Sandeep, is that you don't want to come. See, everybody wants to spend time with their family, but you have to make some sacrifice, too. Until you invest time and energy, how do you expect to make more money?"

I could tell he felt obligated to give me another chance, and for a moment I actually felt sorry for him. I felt undeserving of his patience and saddened that he felt coerced by his friendship with Rajiv to continue to work with me.

"You have to be a little lovey-dovey with patients, Sandeep. Private practice is lovey-dovey. Let's say I adjust the antihypertensive. I will tell the patient to come back in a few days to check the blood pressure. If I am ordering a test, I will tell them to come back to discuss the results."

"Sure, boss," I said, just wanting to get off the phone.

"Look, I am very fair," he said. "You and me should promote together. Let's take out an hour from our busy schedules and meet some physicians in Queens. Once they see us together, maybe some of your brother's friends will start sending us a few patients. If you could get one or two internists who are not sending me patients to start sending you patients—if I can get four or five new patients a month through you who are getting everything done in the office—then it is a plus point. That is all I am asking. I am not asking for a hundred percent of their business."

I told him that I would try to make this happen. When I got off the phone, I felt nauseated. I took a deep breath, and a dry heave welled up in my chest. Water filled my eyes. It was all I could do to keep from vomiting.

THIRTEEN

Deluge

Midway on our life's journey, I found myself
In dark woods, the right road lost. To tell
About those woods is hard—so tangled and rough . . .
　　　　　　—Dante, *The Inferno*, Canto 1,
　　　　　　　　translated by Robert Pinsky

To his credit, Chaudhry did try to make it work. We experimented with different arrangements—seeing patients in Valley Stream, reading echos in Richmond Hill, even doing stress tests on weeknights after I left the hospital—but nothing gelled. For a few months I even went to an office in Harlem, not far from where I lived, where Chaudhry rented space from a jowly, phlegmatic Bangladeshi internist who seemed to think the world of himself. On my first day he gave me a tour of the facility, which occupied the entire second floor of an industrial office building next door to a McDonald's. "You are from India?" he asked with a strong accent.

I nodded, surveying the space, feigning awe. I asked him how long he had been working there.

"You want to know if I am renting?" he said coyly. "That is what you want to know?"

"Yes," I lied.

He took his time answering. "So let us just say we own the whole operation," he said proudly.

It was a huge practice with nearly a dozen employees and a plenitude of patients, mostly Dominican immigrants, who were shuffled through a dense maze of exam rooms. The waiting area always had a loud buzz, a communal conviviality, even at nine o'clock on Saturday morning. Spanish-speaking assistants were available, but they had many duties besides translation, so patients would sometimes wait hours to be seen. There was a podiatrist down the hall who was also renting space. He had an alert, shiny face and a streetwise, almost sinister aura. He would periodically come over, hinting that he wanted referrals, forcing small talk, slowing me down. He kept promising to refer his diabetics to me—as if I needed more patients—but he never did. We set up an echo machine next to my exam room so patients could be scanned while waiting for an interpreter. As soon as one became available, I'd take advantage and quickly go through two or three examinations without a break, slightly decanting the crowded waiting area. If I ordered a stress test, the patient would be offered car service to Chaudhry's office on Long Island, along with a voucher for lunch.

By the end, Chaudhry was treating me like a naive younger brother whom he was merely tolerating. He was clearly dissatisfied with my performance, though technically I was doing everything he was asking of me. Maybe he knew how I felt about his practice—or about private practice in general. At one point he drew up a contract giving me a small portion of the echo and stress fees as an incentive to work harder, but when payday arrived, I was reimbursed according to the old flat-fee formula.

When he finally let me go in the spring of 2008, it was over the phone. "What I am saying, Sandeep, is, you have a shop, you open up a shop, anybody who walks in, you have to have a smiley face, right? These are small things that I hate to tell you, but these things are missing."

I had that sad, strange feeling of being jilted by someone I'd never wanted to be with.

"If the money comes in, I don't mind paying you, but right now you are living on my pie. What I have been trying to do for the last two years is create a separate pie for you, but somehow we have failed."

Unsure of how to respond, I stared at the speakerphone in my office. My leg was jumping up and down like a jackhammer.

"I don't see anybody referring patients to you, Sandeep. Sameer Chawla was sending in January, February, March—and then zero. I want to help you, but in this tight situation at least one patient should be referred to you through some connection. But not a single patient is coming."

"I don't know why Sameer stopped referring," I said. Sameer Chawla was a good friend of Rajiv's. In January, Chaudhry and I had gone to his ramshackle office in Queens Village with a platter of Indian sweets and a few referral pads printed with Chaudhry's contact information and a list of the insurance plans we accepted. We waited cravenly in our white coats among quiet turbaned patients until we were called in to see him. When we finally sat down with him, he seemed friendly enough, and he pledged to lend his support; but the goodwill had lasted only a few months.

"Sandeep, you have to understand, running a big show costs a lot of money," Chaudhry said. "I have two thousand square feet to cover, plus staff, plus nuclear machine, plus echo tech, plus Malik, plus Denis, plus certifications. I am no longer even doing stress tests every Saturday because if only five patients are coming, I still have to give full payment to Denis, full payment for the staff, full day to Malik. If I am not doing ten-plus nuclears on a given day, I am losing money."

My throat was dry. The other line rang, but I ignored it.

"Last Thursday I canceled my office," he went on. "I was sitting down like a CEO and thinking, Hey, Amir, what is going on? Why your revenue is so scanty? Do you know that now I only get thirty dollars for a follow-up and a hundred dollars for a new consult? If we don't order a test—echo, carotid, arterial Doppler, nuclear, or stress echo—well, seeing patients is just garbage."

"But I order those tests," I said weakly.

"I am not talking about you, Sandeep! What I am saying is that in private practice the overhead is so high. And then on top of it I have to pay my biller. I'm telling you honestly, last year I was in debt."

I didn't believe him, but at this point it didn't matter.

"So we can meet with Dr. Richards, like you wanted," I said, trying not to sound desperate. "We can invite Dr. Kapoor out to lunch again."

But it was too late. "Sandeep, I respect you and I love you, but dollar has to come to pay you. If I get nada, then rather we both sit at home on the weekend. I have a family, four kids; living that lifestyle is expensive. If money is not coming, Amir cannot pay you. You have to understand, I am not a hospital."

After hanging up, I felt woozy, so I went outside for some air. I sat down on a bench near the parking lot. In the distance, tulips were shooting out of tiny plots on the sidewalk, like hands coming out of a grave. Chaudhry's admonitions kept echoing through my head. "In private practice, you have to stay busy. If you don't stay busy, you can't make it work." Now what to do? What did this mean? Were we going to default on our apartment? Were we going to have to switch Mohan to the shitty local school? Was I going to have to go back to taking Sonia's father's handouts? Or perhaps worst of all, was I going to have to quit my job and go into private practice full-time? I resolved not to tell Sonia anything, at least not immediately. I was hoping to find more work before we spent down the little savings we'd accrued.

Shortly afterward, Sonia and I went on a long-planned trip with Mohan to Block Island, our first vacation in over a year. I hadn't wanted to go, but I couldn't bring myself to cancel at the last minute. We packed a cooler and a couple of suitcases and drove up to Point Judith, Rhode Island, to catch the ferry. The dock was brimming with summery excitement. Pretty girls in clingy summer dresses were clutching their boyfriends and sipping beer. We were the picture of happiness: a successful Manhattan doctor couple on an exclusive weekend getaway with their four-year-old son. But the picture lied.

The ferry ride was choppy. Halfway across Block Island Sound I was wiping vomit off Mohan's seat. When we arrived on the island, the sky was like a jar of dirty cotton balls. Stormy winds had started to blow. We hailed a cab to our inn. When we pulled up on the gravelly drive, it was already dusk. Whitewashed wood recliners were arrayed randomly on the sloping front lawn. A flock of blackbirds were zigzagging in the distance like one collective organism, apart from a lone straggler trying to merge with the group. Transfixed, I watched them fly overhead.

That night, after unpacking, I went for a run. The rain had stopped, though the trees were still dripping noisily. The path through the field was muddy. The tall grass scraped against my green Gap pants. Because I had stupidly forgotten to bring my sneakers, I was wearing old leather dress shoes that were coming apart at the soles. I sprinted in near pitch darkness, feeling the pasty wetness in my toes. The shadows of trees sliced across the path. The air smelled of manure. My feet were splashing into puddles and crunching on fallen branches. I tripped on a reed, but I kept on going.

Errant thoughts were racing through my head, flitting away like tiny minnows before I could grasp them. What is happening to me? Maybe I am depressed, or perhaps I am going mad; I don't know. I want to regain some control, but the reality is that there is very little one can control in life. I find it hard to accept that, to let things go, to let things be, to see beauty in the obstacles, the denials, the thwarting of your goals and ambitions, to accept things as they are, as having their own kind of beauty and logic.

A strange feeling had settled over me like a film of perspiration. At times it would well up inside me like fluid filling a cavern, and as I would fill up, my neck and shoulders would get tight, and it would flow over my eyes, and that was when I felt most out of control. The fount would gush forth at the most inopportune times, and I could not control it, no matter how hard I tried. Dr. Adams, the psychiatrist I'd been seeing for the past few months, asked me to describe it as I faced him squarely in his tiny office on the Upper West Side.

"It's like butterflies in the belly," I said. "It isn't anger. Perhaps it's anxiety that I cannot express the anger."

"Why the anxiety?"

"I don't know, but I am waking up with it and the workday hasn't even begun. How do I make it stop?"

I had become a slave to my circumstances. Dad was, too, for most of his life, but he didn't experience the anxiety, just the darkness. I used to be so happy when Dad was happy. I didn't want that to be the case for Mohan. I didn't want his happiness to depend on me. I had adopted so many of Dad's traits: paranoia, brooding, reluctant embrace of responsibility, a tendency to blame others for one's own problems. Of course, I took on some good qualities, like commitment and perseverance—but, unfortunately, also self-righteousness, melancholy, insecurity, inflexibility. Recognizing this didn't make it any easier, though. Perhaps what I was grieving over most was the inability to overcome my limitations.

The following day I finally got to spend some one-on-one time with Mohan. "Did you have a good dream or a bad dream?" I asked him when he woke up.

"I had"—he mulled over the answer—"a funny dream! A doggy came to my house. I loved it."

We spent the morning at the inn. The clouds had cleared, and the sun was shining brightly. Mohan and I tossed water balloons on the lawn. We visited a nearby petting farm. We swung together on a hammock strung between two trees.

"I want to go forward, not backward."

"That's forward, too, Mohan. Another forward."

"Another forward?"

"Yes, another forward. You want to try?"

"Uh-kay!"

In the afternoon we went down to Old Harbor and had ice-cream cones while Sonia window-shopped. A band was playing at a tavern across the street. Mohan jiggled in my arms to the music. We watched as the ferry brought in another group of travelers. "It was a bad boat, Dadda," he reminded me. "It was a bad ride!"

That night, as a storm again raged, he settled next to me on a rocking love seat on the porch. Resting on my shoulder, his big head was a weight of stability and contentment. At that moment, nothing else seemed to matter. All the sacrifices in my life seemed worthwhile. I nuzzled him, smudging the lenses of my spectacles. I rubbed my stubbly cheek on his neck and shoulder. He giggled.

"This whole town is a pool," he declared.

"You're right," I said. "That's funny."

We stared into pitch. Water streamed in rivulets off the awning. Flowerpots were swinging wildly as the sky roared, periodically issuing electrical discharges into the blackness. Like me, Mohan seemed to find the storm relaxing. Clutching his hand, I could almost feel it vibrating, as if he were possessed of some otherworldly spirit. I palmed his cranium, squeezing it softly the way my father used to whenever I had a fever. He looked up at me and smiled, his tiny teeth arrayed like two rows of Chiclets. I wanted to be around him every single moment of his life. Marriage, I told myself, is the price of admission to the amusement park that is Mohan.

No doubt our marriage had suffered in the four years since he was born; it had slowly, inexorably turned into an anxious wait to be disappointed. My mind had been going over old issues, old arguments, regurgitating the nasty things that were said, the old irritations. The stress of the financial situation and the moonlighting, adding to the pressure of my regular job and the ongoing guilt of not spending enough time with my patients, my colleagues, or my family, led to a state of chronic edginess and angry outbursts. When I'd come home, I'd feel stressed, unhappy. I didn't want to talk, but it was impossible to avoid interaction in our shoebox apartment. And when I told Sonia any of this, it inevitably led to more conflict. "The way you reacted yesterday with obvious seething anger makes me wonder what good are these sessions with Dr. Adams," she once said.

"What do you want me to say? Tell me what you want me to say, and I'll say it."

"I want to let go of resentments and live in the present moment, Sandeep. I'm being beaten down by all this."

"Can we please stop having these discussions in front of Mohan?"

"What do you want me to do, Sandeep? Mohan, stop it! We are living lives of quiet desperation. I've been trying to tell you, but it doesn't seem to bother you."

I had almost forgotten the way things used to be: the secret smiles, the tenderness. What had happened to those times? Were they a figment of my imagination? Perhaps they were, and the true reality was exposed only after we became parents. I had been a success at everything I'd tried: physics, medicine, fatherhood. Except perhaps at being a husband. But entropy is an inexorable force. It takes two to have a healthy relationship but only one to screw it up.

I was constantly fantasizing about living my life all over again. It felt as if all the big adventures were finished and now I was just running out the clock. I was having dreams that I had never gotten married, never become a doctor or husband or father. I was going through the motions, searching for something, but I didn't know what. No doubt I was following a script. But character is destiny. There is only so much you can do to overcome the constraints of your biology.

On the porch I looked down at Mohan. A tear trickled down the bridge of my nose. Deep love is always mixed with a tinge of sadness because of the constant threat of its evaporating and the knowledge that it is short-lived, that it will all be over one day.

"Dadda, you're sad."

"No, I'm not."

"Yes, you are. You have that sad look on your face."

I forced a smile. "Give me a kiss." He brushed his soft lips gently on my cheek. It tickled.

"Why do you have to go to the office?"

"You know why."

"Why?"

"You know."

"Money?"

I laughed. "Yes."

"So we can have money to buy lunch and clothes and toys?"

I had to smile. "Yeah!"

"But if you need money, you can just go to the bank."

"And if you don't have money in the bank?"

He thought for a moment. "Then you have to sit on a chair or a piece of wood and say"—his voice suddenly got deeper—"'I want some money. Give me some money, please.'"

Again I laughed. "Let's go," I said.

He stood up. "You can't pass unless you answer my riddle," he said. I nodded. He paused for a moment. "What has hair, swings from branch to branch, and goes *ooh ooh ooh ooh?*"

"Monkey?"

"Yes." Lightning crackled. "What's big and strong and stomps like this?" He held out his arm and made a trumpet sound.

"Elephant."

"Right! Okay, what runs fast in the dark and has hair and is really strong and scary?"

"Lion?"

"No."

"Is it a bird or an animal?"

"Animal."

"I give up."

"Monster!"

After putting Mohan to bed, I went to the bathroom. I looked into a mirror, one of those concave reflecting surfaces that magnify your reflection, your flaws and imperfections. I started brushing my teeth. Sonia came in. I still hadn't told her what had happened with Chaudhry (though I did as soon as we returned home). There was a long silence, as if we were trying to think of something to say. Finally she said: "I think we should floss more. It's the next best thing to going to a dentist."

PART III

ADJUSTMENT

FOURTEEN

Deception

We don't want to admit that we are fundamentally dishonest about reality, that we do not really control our own lives.

—Ernest Becker, *The Denial of Death*, 1973

There is one thing that is liberating about middle age. Time is limited. You're old enough to realize that life is finite but still young enough to act on that knowledge. But how to make the most of the time you are allotted? How do you find meaning in an existence you know is going to end? If life is a guaranteed tragedy, what prevents us from sinking into hopelessness, whiling away our time till our time comes?

Perhaps it's children. For many of us, children are our legacy, and what are we striving to do in this world more than bequeathing a piece of ourselves? The anthropologist Ernest Becker argues that anxiety over death is the most powerful force affecting human behavior. He says we deny our certain mortality by accruing symbolic victories of enduring value: conquering an empire, building a temple, writing a book. We strive for heroism as a means of denying our eventual fate. And in the vast array of possible immortality projects, perhaps none is as powerful as having children. Kids help you learn to accept your mortality because you start to love something more than yourself. Our selfishness consumes us. Children can rescue us from this fate.

In many ways my children have been the redeeming grace of my middle years thus far. They are the reason I've compromised and also my salvation from the distress of compromise.

———

When I finally told Rajiv that Chaudhry had let me go, he of course blamed me. "You should have listened," he said sadly. "It was easy money. Now what the hell are you going to do?"

We were sitting in my office with the door closed. I yawned, trying to feign a lack of concern, but in reality I was petrified. The savings that Sonia and I had put away from the past two years of moonlighting were dwindling rapidly, and we were expecting our second child to boot. "I could try talking to him again," I said. "I could go to Richmond Hill on Sundays when he doesn't want to work."

"He's not going to take you back," Rajiv barked, obviously frustrated. He didn't need to remind me that the hospital had been providing malpractice coverage for my work with Chaudhry. Now, if I were going to moonlight someplace else, I'd have to purchase my own part-time policy—roughly $17,000 a year—which I couldn't afford. Perhaps the best option now, Rajiv suggested, was to do private practice full-time. Before I could respond, his mobile phone rang. "Hello! Rajiv!" He listened for a few seconds. "Oh, yes, boss," he said pleasantly. "How are you, boss?" Then he stood up and walked out.

Feeling desperate, I phoned Malik, the physician who performed Chaudhry's treadmill tests. By then I had learned that Malik, though occasionally helpful, was a bit of a con artist. He had earned a medical degree in Pakistan but hadn't passed the American board exams, so he wasn't certified to practice independently (that was why he was working for Chaudhry and other physicians). He possessed a sort of worldly weariness, an international playboy charm masquerading as sincerity. He always said yes in the moment, deciding to worry later about the consequences of false promises. Like a politician, he rarely answered the question you posed, just the one he wanted to answer. But one often continues a farce for the sake of a friendship.

"You have to learn how to play the game," Malik told me, trying to explain how I could get back into Chaudhry's good graces. "Your brother knows how to play the game. When he's with a Muslim, he says *salaam alaikum*. When he sees a Sikh, he says *sat sri akal*. Rajiv, Amir, they understand that medicine has become a business. You have to be friendly to have a chance to be successful."

"I'm not friendly?" I blurted out, sounding pathetic even to myself.

"No, you're friendly," Malik said, though I could tell he was lying. "It just takes you time to open up."

I heard him starting the treadmill. "You have to meet Amir face-to-face," he said, as the heavy pounding of a patient's feet began to reverberate in my earpiece. "Ask him what you need to change so you can go back to working every other Saturday. See, you don't know how to manipulate a situation. If he asks you why internists are not sending you patients, appeal to his ego. Tell him, 'They don't want to send us patients because they are jealous of you.'"

I figured anything, even groveling, was worth a try. "So how is Amir's office running without me?" I asked tentatively.

"It's busy," Malik replied. "He is looking to hire someone, even though he still has Ali," the physician's assistant.

"What about the echos?"

"Still piled up on his desk. He reads at night. He goes in on weekends. But a lot of the time he's behind."

That Chaudhry's office was operating a bit less smoothly without me was a small but tangible satisfaction. I heard the treadmill speeding up. "So call him," Malik said. "You have nothing to lose. Remember, he is your brother's best friend."

I phoned Chaudhry the following day. I wanted to meet in person, so he invited me to his home on Long Island. I drove there on a Saturday afternoon in the early summer. It was a stately house in Oyster Bay with manicured lawns and a pool and a tennis court about a mile from where Rajiv lived. I parked in the semicircular driveway. Giant gargoyle planters adorned the front porch. His eldest daughter let me in. Waiting in the ornate foyer while she went to get her father, I noticed a wooden plaque inscribed with gold Arabic letters. Underneath was written: "Even if you don't understand them, these words will ease your daily stress and bring additional income from unknown sources."

Chaudhry greeted me warmly and took me into the living room. He looked relaxed in shorts and a polo shirt. We sat opposite each other, a glass coffee table between us. My heart was beating so hard that my glasses were oscillating on the bridge of my nose. I started to explain my situation, leaning forward, palms open, in a pose of supplication, but before I could get very far, he quickly and mercifully terminated the conversation.

"Sandeep, you were always late," he said with the condescending sympathy of an ex-girlfriend explaining why she'd broken up with you. "Ten, fifteen minutes is okay, but one hour? The girls came to me and said, 'We cannot work with Dr. Jauhar anymore. The patients are coming to the front desk and cursing us.' No offense to you, my friend, but I don't think you are cut out for private practice."

"I am a flawed person," I said lamely, realizing full well that I had probably sabotaged the arrangement from the beginning—going late to the office, complaining about the work, not searching hard for new referrals.

"That's fine, Sandeep," he said, shrugging, "but this is my bread and butter."

"It's my bread and butter, too, Amir. I can't pay my bills without it."

"No," he said, "you have a secure job at the hospital. This practice is all I have, and I have to protect it."

The best he would offer is that I could take more of his doc-of-the-day ER calls. He'd continue to pay me a modest flat fee to answer all his pages and admit all cardiac patients from the ER on a given night who did not already have a cardiologist. As per routine, he would bill and collect all the revenue. He promised to give me a few echos to read, too. It wasn't a lot—much less than I'd hoped for—but with no leverage to negotiate, I quietly accepted the proposal. With another baby on the way and little in the bank, I had no other choice. For me it was a stay of execution.

———

"Mom, these tuna balls are cold! They have to be cooked through, Mohan can't eat these. Mohan, stop it! Do you want mac 'n' cheese? Oh God, the clothes are still wet! Only put a little bit of cheese, Mom, not the whole thing! Mohan, we're making you mac 'n' cheese, so delicious, do you want it? Sandeep, honey, I've got to go!" And then an abrupt click.

Our home life was increasingly frenzied as we prepared for another baby. We talked about putting up a partition to section a small nursery off the master bedroom, but we quickly abandoned the idea. Gerrymandering our tiny apartment wasn't going to solve our space problem. I felt strangely aloof from all the planning. I wasn't sure I even wanted another child, and the prospect of paying a second school tuition in three years filled me with dread. Vegetating in front of television sitcoms at night, I'd see reminders of the deficiencies in my life, accentuating my restlessness. For months the only reliable pleasure—transient, empty—was a quick masturbation or a late-night smoke.

Sonia insisted we needed more spirituality in our lives, so we spent a few Sunday mornings at the Self-Realization Fellowship Center on Twenty-eighth Street. Mohan would sit between us in the chapel, where huge wooden *oms* and stained glass graced the walls. We'd listen quietly to sermons or to a tone-deaf choir crooning "I Will Sing Thy Name." Everyone at these gatherings spoke softly, deliberately, exuding inner peace (or perhaps cognitive delay). SRF was founded by Paramahansa Yogananda, the Indian guru who moved to California in the 1920s and popularized kriya meditation and yoga with his *Autobiography of a Yogi*. In the book, Yogananda writes that "one half-minute of kriya equals one year of natural spiritual unfoldment." Sonia and I tried it a few times, but yoga provided little respite from our ceaseless bickering—over money, over whether (and where) we should move. (She wanted to go to New Jersey to be near her parents; I wanted to be on Long Island, closer to my work.) "You're so smart, and what did it get us?" she cried out in a weak and tearful moment. "You have a Ph.D. in physics, for God's sake! You should have done finance or derivatives."

I, too, was prone to fits of temper, as though my neural circuitry had been pruned to ferry stimuli directly to my amygdala, bypassing reason. Once, I found myself yelling at Terence, the guy answering the phone at Asphalt Green, where Mohan took swim classes on Saturday mornings. I'd been unable to register Mohan online for the new semester. I had called the front office the day before but had gotten the runaround. The woman on the phone had been unable to confirm that Mohan was signed up because the computer was down. She said she'd call me back, but she never did. The following day, Terence tried to patch me through to Lewis, the regular guy, but when he couldn't, I just lost it.

"I've spent hundreds of dollars at your school, and no one calls me back!" I screamed into the phone. "I'm going to report you to the administration! I spent an hour on the phone yesterday"—an exaggeration—"and I can't do this anymore!"

"What do you want done?" Terence asked calmly.

"I want my son signed up for Super Sprites, not Dancing Dolphins, on Saturdays at nine-thirty!" I bellowed. And then I faltered, terribly flustered. It sounded ridiculous, even to me. For a moment there was silence.

"Okay, Doctor, I'll take care of it," he said sympathetically.

For a few moments I didn't say anything. Finally, I said evenly, "His name is Mohan. Last semester he was in Dancing Dolphins, but this—"

"Yes, I know. I'll take care of it. You'll get a confirmation e-mail in a few minutes."

I took a deep breath, and my eyes watered with relief. "Thank you, Terence," I whispered.

———

With the additional doc-of-the-day calls, my life became even more hectic. Every Monday I'd typically get paged all night long. On the phone I'd take down the names of patients being admitted to me and discuss a rudimentary treatment strategy with the ER. Then, early Tuesday morning, prior to starting my regular workday, skipping breakfast and groggy from lack of sleep, I'd rush to the hospital to see the dozen or so patients who'd been assigned to me the night before. The diagnoses were always the same: chest pain, shortness of breath, syncope. Syncope, or fainting, was the most common.

When people stand up, about half a quart of blood initially pools in the legs. This decreases blood flow to the heart and brain, and that would make you faint if it weren't for a chain of reflexes that kick into action. Adrenaline is released, which speeds up the heart and increases its pumping force. It also tightens up the blood vessels to force the blood northward, most importantly to the brain. The net effect is that when you stand up, you stay up.

For reasons we don't understand, this response can go awry. The adrenaline surge can lead to vigorous contractions of a heart that doesn't have much blood in it. The body is fooled into thinking it is physiologically overexcited, so the heart slows down, blood vessels relax, blood flow to the brain drops, and eventually so does the body.

The common faint was enshrined in my adolescent imagination by movies. Remember the beautiful heroine—fainters on film are always women—overcome by shock, touching her brow with the back of her hand, and falling limply into waiting arms? Her faint was stereotyped and contrived—yet riveting. It made fainting seem benign, almost glamorous.

But in the ER, syncope was a decidedly less romantic disease. "Syncopizers"—often elderly patients on multiple medications—were some of the most dreaded patients I saw on my postcall days because I never knew what to do with them. Send them home and I'd worry they'd drop dead from an arrhythmia. Admit them to the hospital and I'd think of all the money being wasted on a most certainly useless diagnostic workup—EKG monitoring, echo, head CT, etc.—that would provide an answer less than 20 percent of the time. (Yet out of fear of missing something, I'd almost always order it.) "Gomers go to ground"— old people tend to fall—was a maxim from residency. Did every demented octogenarian who'd fallen really need to be admitted to the hospital?

Mrs. Hines had an egg-shaped welt on her forehead and two black eyes, like a raccoon's, the result of a flop on her kitchen floor. She was in her late eighties, carried a diagnosis of dementia, and took about twelve different medications, including two that can cause orthostatic hypotension, in which blood pressure drops precipitously on standing. "I'm going to take her home," her husband said when I went to see her in the ER in the very early morning. "She doesn't need to be here."

"Then why did you bring her in?" I said, barely suppressing a yawn and thinking ahead to the seven other patients I had to see: Eleanor Murphy, also with syncope; Jose Ruiz, two days of left leg numbness, cardiac enzymes borderline positive; Fumaria Raghavan, shortness of breath and palpitations for three days, now with slurred speech . . .

"I don't know," Mr. Hines replied, nonplussed. "Home attendant told me to. I made a mistake."

She was lying on a stretcher, her hands clasped across her chest. She appeared disoriented. "My toes are broken," she said. "A bar of wood fell from the shed."

"I was told you fell in your kitchen, ma'am," I said.

Momentarily, she looked perplexed. "No, it was out in the fields, I think. I was with people. They didn't tell me not to be there."

I examined her digits. "Your toes don't look broken to me."

"Yes, they're okay now. See, I can wiggle them."

I took out my stethoscope. I asked her if she felt dizzy. She said no.

"Have you ever gotten dizzy?"

"No."

"Are you sure?"

"Yes, I'm sure."

"I was told you came in because you were dizzy."

She thought for a moment. "Yes, I get dizzy sometimes, but only after I fall."

Dizzy from a lack of sleep, I felt like falling over myself. There was no doubt that after such a traumatic spill she would have to be admitted. I slipped my stethoscope under her gown. After a few seconds she pushed me away. "That's it, no more, no more."

"Excuse me?"

"No more freebies, sonny."

"I'm sorry?"

"You know, feeling me up. Getting something for nothing."

I had to laugh. "I just need to examine you, ma'am."

"I'm not sick!"

"Then why are you in the hospital?"

"I like to come to the hospital," she replied. "There are smart people here. Good people, bad people, dumb people."

I helped her sit up so she could dangle her legs. I was trying to reproduce her symptoms by causing blood to pool in her lower extremities, setting off the fainting cascade. If she didn't feel any symptoms or if her blood pressure didn't drop, I was going to stand her up to stress her even more.

It didn't get that far, though. After less than a minute of sitting, she said she was faint and closed her eyes. When I checked her blood pressure, it had dropped fifty points. The test was positive; we could stop. I tried to tell her, but she was already out. I called for a nurse and moved on to my next patient.

With so many patients to see after a call night, things would sometimes get mixed up. I remember one patient, Ajit Singh, a Sikh man with congestive heart failure who was about to be started on dialysis. He was sporting a red turban and a long white beard, tied into small knots. "Do you get short of breath?" I asked him in Punjabi, thumbing through his chart.

He nodded. The chart said he had renal failure, a consequence of his heart disease. There was a plan to place a catheter in his arm to start dialysis, but when I mentioned this to him, he pretended to know nothing about it. I pointed to his wrist, where the fistula would go in. Yes, he said, they had put a needle in his vein not long ago, some test. I explained to him that this was a sign that his kidneys were about to fail and that he would have to be hooked up to a machine to clean his blood three times a week. He stared at me, in shock.

A nurse walked in. "Mr. Singh is in the other bed," she said. I'd been talking to the wrong patient!—though one who also had heart failure. (The nurses often roomed patients with the same diagnosis together.)

Fool! I screamed into my head. I quickly explained my mistake and apologized. Instead of being upset, the patient was effusive. "Thank you, thank you," he said in Punjabi, clasping his hands together and obviously relieved. "Next only to God is the doctor."

My doc-of-the-day patients were often frustrating to manage, and not just because of the volume. A big reason was their limited resources. They rarely saw a doctor regularly, and poverty and lack of health insurance or social support were constant stressors in their lives. A social worker on one of my cases told me that for most patients, domestic problems or destructive habits were entrenched. There was little that could be done for them in the hospital, and patients were often lost to followup after discharge. She did the best she could, but there was only so much that could be done. Though she was trained as a clinical psychologist, most of her work revolved around mundane issues like insurance forms and discharge planning.

Juana Morales, in her late thirties, was writhing when I first met her: mouth foaming; teeth clenched; in severe abdominal pain, which a cardiac catheterization confirmed was due to heart failure compromising blood flow to her gut. A blue plastic tube was feeding oxygen to a pressurized ventilation mask that was strapped tightly to her face. A nurse was at the bedside, adjusting the oxygen. "What do you want me to do?" she asked me impatiently. "Morphine, Lasix, albuterol, what?"

"Let's try Lasix first," I replied.

"*Caliente, muy caliente*," the patient cried when her mask was briefly taken off, complaining about the temperature in the room. Her husband was with her, along with their eight-year-old son. They were from Ecuador. Father and son looked alike, sporting dark hair spiked with gel and pressed Le Tigre shirts and crisp blue jeans. Her husband demanded to know why we couldn't adjust the air-conditioning for his wife. "The heat is not good for her," he cried. "She can't breathe." I told him I would request that the thermostat be adjusted, but that her shortness of breath was due to heart failure, not the temperature in the room. She would require intravenous medications to relieve her symptoms.

She had no health insurance, though the chart stated that her husband did. I asked him if she had a green card. Immigration status was going to be very relevant in deciding how we were going to manage her. As a cardiology fellow at NYU, I had treated several illegal immigrants with end-stage heart failure. Usually there were hospitals in their native countries that performed heart transplants, but if they went back home, they would not be allowed to return to America, so they almost never wanted to discuss that option. (And none of them could afford transplants in their native lands anyway.) In many cases, the only hope for an illegal immigrant with end-stage heart failure was to raise the quarter of a million dollars for a cardiac transplant herself.

Her husband didn't answer my question about her status. "It is essential that you tell us everything," I urged. "The only people who will know are those who need to know."

Then he said, "No, she is illegal."

My heart sank. "This is a problem," I said. "It is going to be very difficult to get your wife a new heart, and that is probably what she needs to live."

He seemed genuinely shocked. "You just let them die?" he said.

Now it was my turn to waver. "In some cases they do die because there are so few hearts available," I said carefully. "There are only about two hundred heart transplants per year in New York City. And that is in a city of eight million people."

He turned away. "Don't worry about her immigration status," I said. "We won't tell anyone."

"I don't care about that," he replied. "I just care about my wife. I want her to live." His lips quivered, and tears started to fall from his eyes. He excused himself and stepped into the hallway. Their son was watching quietly. His big brown eyes looked awful, scared and confused about what was happening, why his father was crying. I was sure he would re-member this moment for the rest of his life.

The nurse stepped outside to comfort the husband. She returned two minutes later. "He says he is illegal, too," she said.

Juana Morales wasn't the only patient who was not forthcoming about the reality of her life. Ellie McGlone was a college student in her early twenties with red hair, pretty features, and a disarming sincerity. When I first met her in the ER, she told me that she had been on a KLM flight from Helsinki, Finland, to Detroit, where her grandmother lived, when she developed palpitations and dizziness. Finding her pale and sweaty, a flight attendant had taken her to the back of the plane to lie down. An EKG monitor applied to her chest, she said, revealed ven-tricular tachycardia, a potentially life-threatening arrhythmia.

When the plane landed at La Guardia Airport for a short layover, she hailed a taxi and asked the driver to take her to the nearest hospital. The airline had arranged for an ambulance, but she had refused it. "They wanted three paramedics in the ambulance instead of two," she explained. "I don't have that kind of money." I told her that given the na-ture of the emergency, she would not have been responsible for the charges. "See, I didn't know that," she replied matter-of-factly.

She went to Flushing Hospital Medical Center because that was where the taxi driver took his own family when they were sick. Doctors there, after hearing her history, inserted a central intravenous line below her collarbone. They gave her some medications to stabilize her heart-beat, monitored her for several hours, and then transferred her to LIJ for further evaluation.

I asked about her medical history. She told me that her family suf-fered from an unknown blood disorder that caused premature heart at-tacks. Her mother had died at age thirty-three. Three maternal uncles had died in their thirties and forties. All her cousins were dead. The first, Sarah, died at age eighteen; Sarah's brother, at age twenty-two. John, Josh, and Matthew all died in their twenties. Apart from her grandmother, my patient was the last one in her immediate family who was still alive.

I inquired about the medical workup in Finland. She told me she'd had a heart attack in her early twenties, necessitating angioplasty of a major coronary artery. When I asked for permission to obtain medical records from hospitals in Helsinki, she refused. "There are confidentiality issues," she explained.

I performed a physical exam. Her blood pressure was 120/80: normal. Her lungs sounded clear, and her heartbeat was regular and normal. I noticed a long scar along the right side of her back, where, she told me, she had previously had lung surgery. "A blood clot was choking off part of my lung," she explained, another consequence of the blood disorder.

An EKG and an echocardiogram were performed: both normal. Continuous EKG monitoring was normal. Routine blood tests revealed nothing unusual. Though she said she had been taking digitalis, the drug was undetectable in her blood.

I asked if there were family members I could talk to. There were some distant relations in Finland, but she didn't want me to contact them. The same went for her fiancé in Washington, D.C., who had weathered "enough stress" because of her many hospitalizations. There was a phone number for her grandmother in the front of the chart, but she insisted that no one call her. "She buried nine children!" my patient cried. "She has suffered enough."

Because of the central line in her chest, she had been requesting painkillers, mostly morphine, around the clock. She had also been complaining of nausea but had refused to take Zofran, the usual antiemetic, instead requesting promethazine, which accentuates the effect of morphine. "It is classic drug-seeking behavior," a nurse told me.

I didn't know what to do, so we waited to get more information. That evening her grandmother phoned the on-call resident, who had left a voice mail for her earlier in the day. "Oh, the old clotting disorder story," the grandmother said. She explained that her granddaughter had used this story many times before to get hospitalized.

I felt sorry for my patient—but angry, too, at the lie. When I told her that we would no longer give her narcotics, she demanded to be discharged immediately. I tried to get her to stay until we could figure out what to do for her, but she left about an hour later, after the central line had been removed from her chest. "People don't know what it's like to lose your whole family, your mother, your cousins, and then be the last one and have to keep on living," she said on her way out.

Deception by patients assumes many different guises. One is what the diagnostic bible of psychiatry calls malingering: "the intentional production of false or grossly exaggerated physical or psychiatric symptoms" motivated by the desire to avoid work, evade prosecution, obtain drugs, and so on. Another, spurred by the need to play the role of a sick person, is termed factitious disorder. When patients lie to themselves, convincing themselves that they are sick when they are not, the condition is called somatization disorder. And of course there is plain evasion, when patients like Ms. Morales simply withhold the truth about key details of their lives.

I believe Ellie was probably suffering from a malignant form of factitious disorder called Munchausen syndrome. In this syndrome, patients will often intentionally produce or distort symptoms because of a need to be seen as ill or injured. They will undergo painful tests or diagnostic procedures if necessary to maintain the lie.

"Deception" is a charged word when used in the context of medicine. It encapsulates precisely what we dread most in a doctor-patient relationship, which should be founded on trust, honesty, and openness. And yet it is there in the medical profession, and it often runs both ways. We physicians deceive our patients, too. We don't always reveal when we make mistakes. We order unnecessary tests. We mislead by maintaining that our therapies (the placebo injections from my grandfather's era, for example, and much of spinal surgery or angioplasty today) have more value, more evidence behind them, than they actually do. And we deceive ourselves, too. We espouse the patriotic (but deeply misguided) notion that the American medical system is the best in the world. We deny the sickness in our system and the role we as a profession have played in creating that sickness. We obsessively push ourselves to do more and more, for reasons, both knightly and knavish, that we often hide from ourselves.

Though I have thought deeply about these issues for much of my career, I am not immune to this sort of masquerade. I have at times practiced a sort of ethics of double effect. I have lied to myself and to my patients in the service of a larger goal.

In the summer of 2006 I met Lily Dunhill, an eighty-eight-year-old lady (in every sense of the word) with a severely leaky heart valve that was constantly putting her into acute heart failure. She wore a powdered face, thick lipstick, and salon-done blondish hair sitting on bony, wasted temples. When I first encountered her in the emergency room about a year before she died, I asked her with whom she lived. She told me her mother.

"No, seriously," I said.

"My mother," she insisted.

"Come on, how old are you?"

She grinned slyly. "Old enough to get married."

She became one of my most beloved patients, coming to see John and me every few weeks. We admired her no-nonsense yet playful approach to life. "See, I'm direct," she once told us. "I'm not going to tell you one thing when it's another. You know who taught me how to smoke? It was during the war. It was a group of girls. So one time they said, 'C'mon, Lily, just smoke,' and that got the ball rolling, and now I can't breathe."

Though I generally do not practice primary care, I didn't want Lily to have to travel to see multiple doctors, so I agreed to serve as her general physician as well as her cardiologist. She'd call John or me several times a week to update us on her condition (or sometimes just to chat). So it came as a shock when we learned one afternoon that she was in the intensive care unit. A few days earlier, she had been brought in by ambulance to the emergency room, where she'd had a respiratory arrest. She had been intubated with a breathing tube and admitted to the ICU with a diagnosis of worsening kidney and heart failure, under the care of Dr. Charles Muller, a critical care specialist. John rushed over to see her but was told by the ICU team that it was managing her case and "did not need cardiology input." I went to see her anyway and made several treatment recommendations, which the ICU team did not follow.

John and I went to the ICU for three straight days. Though she was sedated and breathing with the aid of a ventilator, her lips curled upward in a smile whenever she saw us. Her skin was jaundiced, the color of polenta, a sign of liver failure. She had kidney failure, too, and had stopped making urine. On the third day I took a senior resident aside and asked him why the team hadn't checked liver function tests. He said that Dr. Muller did not want her LFTs checked. "But what's the etiology of her liver failure?" I demanded. He said that he did not know and that I should discuss it with Dr. Muller.

"I've been an ICU resident, too," I said, getting angry. "You're taking care of the sickest patients in the hospital, but that doesn't mean you shouldn't listen to a patient's doctor. Our input should have some bearing on this case." He again told me to discuss my concerns with Dr. Muller. "Fine," I said. "Take me to him."

Muller was sitting in his office, working on his desktop. He was a short man in his late forties with a full head of bushy salt-and-pepper hair. I stood in the doorway, with John and the resident waiting behind me. "I'd like to talk with you about my patient, Lily Dunhill," I said. He looked up, as if he'd been expecting me. I told him I was concerned about her kidney failure. Was she going to be dialyzed? He said no. I asked why not.

"It isn't appropriate," Muller replied, "and Dr. Haney, the nephrologist, agrees with me." He said he had inserted a catheter in her pulmonary artery, which showed that her cardiac output was severely compromised and that the blood pressure in her lungs was alarmingly high. "She has severe mitral valve regurgitation," Muller reminded me. "That's not going to get any better."

"Why is she jaundiced?" I demanded. "Why not check her LFTs?"

"What am I going to do with the information?" Muller retorted. "She is at the end of her life. I could dialyze her, but for what purpose?"

"So that decision has already been made?"

"Yes, absolutely. As a doctor I don't have to present every option to my patient. I can act with discretion."

"She's a sentient human being," I cried. "She has the right to know if you've written her off. If you're withholding potentially lifesaving treatment, she needs to know about it."

Muller nearly jumped out of his seat. "Hold on, Dr. Jauhar. I don't understand what you're saying, so maybe you could explain!"

"Look, I respect your clinical judgment," I said, backing down a bit, "but these decisions aren't made in a vacuum. Whether you're withholding or withdrawing treatment, she needs to be a party to that decision."

"Dr. Jauhar, with all due respect, I don't want her LFTs checked. I absolutely do not want dialysis discussed with her. If you want her managed differently, you can take her to the CCU under your care. I'm not suggesting you do that, by the way," he quickly added.

"Why shouldn't she know?" I shouted, giving up any attempt to hold a civil conversation.

"Because even if she said yes, I still wouldn't offer her dialysis. It would be futile and inappropriate."

I pressed him. "What about trying to wean her off the ventilator?"

"I can't wean the ventilator with that chest X-ray. Plus, she can't come off the ventilator if she isn't making urine. She'll drown in her own fluids."

He assured me that all decisions had been discussed with her son.

"But she doesn't lack capacity," I said. "She doesn't need a surrogate. She can make decisions for herself."

I stormed back to my office. I didn't know what to think. Was my judgment being blinded by sentiment? Was I trying too hard to save Lily, or was Muller not trying hard enough?

The following day I went to speak to Dr. Lerner, the chairman of the department of medicine. "It's unfortunate," he told me in his spacious office after I had delivered my complaint.

I said that it showed a certain—I fumbled for the right word—"I don't know, arrogance, insecurity . . ."

"It's not arrogance," Lerner said. He told me how when he was in the ICU as a patient, his primary care physician had come by, but no one had followed his recommendations either. "I found it kind of strange, but I've seen this attitude in many ICU doctors. Muller doesn't like to be questioned. I've seen him go down a certain path and be very reluctant to change. Maybe it is insecurity." He suggested that I transfer my patient to the cardiac unit and take care of her myself.

The next morning, as transfer preparations were being made, I went to see Lily. Muller and his team were at her bedside. All I caught was "and I think it's inappropriate," and then they went on to the next patient.

When I walked into Lily's room, she was on her side, being cleaned. A tube was in her rectum, draining liquid stool. I told the nurse that I was going to take her to the CCU. The nurse appeared relieved.

Predictably, Lily's sojourn in the CCU was a disaster. She was unable to be weaned from the ventilator. Her liver failure worsened. Even as it became clear to me that she was going to die and that my aggressive interventions had been for no good purpose, I became very reluctant to change course, too. We checked blood tests several times per day. I inserted a pressure catheter in her pulmonary artery to monitor her hemodynamics. I started her on continuous veno-venous hemodialysis, but the dialysis catheter repeatedly got clotted because of her low blood pressure. The breathing tube remained in her throat till the end. Eventually she succumbed to multisystem organ failure and sepsis, nearly a week after I'd transferred her to my care. She was eighty-nine.

At their core, my actions were also a kind of deception: convincing myself, despite all the evidence, that I could save her, stay the inexorable course of her disease. Perhaps I was afraid of failure or embarrassed by my impotence, or maybe I was unwilling to face the grief over a dear patient's dying; I don't know. Those last few days of her life, she almost ceased to be a person for me. She became an experiment, a puzzle, one that I desperately wanted to solve. Of course, I thought of James Irey, the Trinidadian man whom I'd convinced to undergo a cardiac catheterization against his better judgment and who died from complications of the procedure. How much—and how little—had changed in the past four years.

In the end, we all practice a certain amount of deception to make it through our lives. We erect defenses to cope with our deepest fears: of powerlessness, loss, and death. Ernest Becker writes about the "vital lie" that keeps us from facing the true reality of our existence. "We don't want to admit that we do not stand alone, that we always rely on something that transcends us, some system of ideas and powers in which we are embedded." And when that system, personal or professional, fails us, and the anxiety of our existence rushes in, sometimes the best we can do is to simply absorb ourselves in our everyday pursuits. Perhaps this is the solution to medicine's midlife crisis, too: doctors focusing on their noble craft, their relationships with patients, the stuff over which we have some control. Ultimately, this may be the best hope for our professional salvation.

FIFTEEN

Ticktock

Death is not an event in life.   —Ludwig Wittgenstein

That summer, Mohan and I went to Fargo, North Dakota, to celebrate my father's seventieth birthday. (Sonia, understandably nervous given the complications of the last pregnancy, stayed behind in New York.) "Don't fly first-class," my father said when I told him we were coming, though such an extravagance hadn't even occurred to me. "I want my grandson to be strong, learn how to struggle."

"Dad, he's four years old!"

"Still, you don't want to spoil him. It's never too early to teach him right from wrong."

Descending into Fargo on a small commuter jet, I peered out the window at the flat landscape. The fields were barren, dotted with lonely lights. My parents picked us up at the airport. My mother was dressed in an overcoat, though the weather was temperate. My father, insisting on carrying my luggage, struggled with the heavy suitcase. The cuffs on his pants were threadbare. His hair was whiter and more flyaway than I remembered from the last time I'd seen him. He offered me the car keys. On the way home, he was in an inexplicably foul mood.

"Your mother killed herself all week," he groused. "I mean, chicken, fish, gulab jamun, ras malai. It was a bit ridiculous."

"She hasn't seen me in almost a year, Dad."

"Drive with two hands," he ordered. I grudgingly placed my right hand on the steering wheel. My father looked back at my mother. "He still acts like a kid," he said. "He still drives like it's a game."

At the house, I noticed there was rust on the garage girders. Lightbulbs needed to be replaced. One of the kitchen tiles was cracked, and soap dispensers were empty. The house, like my parents, was in a state of subtle decay.

I unpacked my suitcase in the guest room. On the bedside table were some pictures of me from high school, along with a couple of old tennis trophies and my tattered copy of *Zen and the Art of Motorcycle Maintenance.* Inside the closet I noticed the world globe I had used in middle school, as well as my dad's old Petri camera. Each object was heavily laden with memories: the lemon drops my father offered whenever he drove me to school board meetings; the tennis racket I played with when my father forced me to give up my spot on the local team going to the California Interscholastic Federation tennis tournament because Rajiv, whom I had beaten in the qualifying match, was a senior and it was his last opportunity to play CIF. Despite the ambivalent remembrances, the room had a cobbled-together quality, as if it were being used for storage.

Downstairs, my father was sitting at the dining table, sorting through bills. He seemed blank, anxious, worked up. We quietly ate the meal my mother had prepared. My father asked how my work with Chaudhry was going. I hadn't told him much about what had transpired, other than that Chaudhry had cut back on some of my hours. "Sometimes he doesn't give me work, and then I'm short paying my bills," I said offhandedly.

"Does he pay you on time?"

"Yes, he pays," I said, trying to squelch the conversation. "He's not that bad, just a bit stingy with the work."

After dinner we lit candles and cut a small cake. Mohan belted out "Happy Birthday," trying to infuse some celebration into the proceedings. While I went upstairs to put him to bed, my parents cleaned up. Coming back downstairs, I spied my father fishing a birthday envelope out of the trash bin. It was covered in grease and cream. He passed it to my mother. "Keep it," he said. "For a memory."

My sister and her kids arrived the following day. The cousins played hide-and-seek in the backyard. We went go-karting at an amusement park. Every evening after dinner we'd go for ice cream. One evening we went to my father's lab to check out his new microscope. Afterward, in the greenhouse where he grew his wheat hybrids, he tried to explain genetics to Mohan. "What's inside cells?" my father asked him.

"Genes," Mohan replied proudly, as I'd taught him.

"No, chromosomes," my father said sharply. Mohan looked at me, deflated. "You have forty-six chromosomes," my father said.

"Chromosomes have genes in them," I gently explained to Mohan.

"A cell doesn't have genes?" Mohan asked.

"No!" my father barked. "Well, it does, but you can't see them."

Now Mohan was really confused. "The genes are inside chromosomes," I explained. I picked him up. "Do you have to make it so difficult?" I snapped at my father. Turning to Mohan, I said, "Every cell in the body has forty-six chromosomes. Nana has forty-six, Mama has forty-six, you have forty-six, I have forty-six—"

"If you have more or less—forty-five or forty-seven—you will be abnormal!" my father boomed.

My father got increasingly testy as the week wore on. "I don't know what will happen to us," he said in one especially malevolent altercation at the kitchen table. "When you get old, you lose your importance."

"That's the way of the world, Dad," I said evenly, refusing to be emotionally manipulated. "What makes you think our family is any different?"

"I took care of my mother. She died in my arms."

"She died in a nursing home!"

"We visited her three times a day!"

I laughed mirthlessly. I didn't want to continue the argument, but I couldn't stop it either.

"You people don't respect your parents. When we are old . . ." His voice trailed off. "I don't want to see it." He looked sharply at my mother. "I can't believe these kids. I never yelled at my father."

"That's because he died when you were thirteen years old," I said viciously.

Though seventy years old now, he was still the same: inflexible, restless, a victim of his own expectations. There was no question in my mind that he'd wanted us to come for his birthday, and he was probably touched by the gesture, too—even if he couldn't show it—but I couldn't help but think that for him it was more about the ritual of the visit than the sentiment. We were following the same old script from when I was growing up, unable to modify it to cope with the changing times.

"Things are never perfect," I said to my sister when we took a walk around the neighborhood one evening. The air was warm and stale; the sidewalks were empty. Fireflies were starting to light up in the dusky haze. "I was so looking forward to this trip, but things are never perfect."

She strolled beside me but didn't say anything.

"I get so irritated," I said. "I know I shouldn't. I hate myself for it. But if I don't react, it's like I've given up."

"Our parents are probably only going to be around for a few more years," she said softly. "We keep forgetting that."

"I know," I said. I remembered what a doctor friend had told me at the funeral of a colleague's mother. "It's really something to lose your parents," he'd said. "You grow up after you lose your parents." I shook my head to banish the thought. Then I said defiantly to my sister: "I know he's never going to change. But neither am I."

———

Back in New York, I was feeling increasingly weighed down by my bland responsibilities. Everything I was doing—as a doctor, husband, or father—seemed a crude and subpar approximation of what was good and ideal. I kept telling myself to be a witness and observe it all. But experiences refract aberrantly through the haze of gloom. A stick underwater gives the illusion of being bent.

In the fall I impulsively wrote an essay for *The New York Times* about the problem of overtesting in medicine that predictably created a backlash. After the article was published, a group of private cardiologists wrote a letter to my division chief saying they were "outraged . . . We take great offense to the portrayal of medicine on Long Island . . . as being driven solely by money," they wrote. "Although you can argue that there are a few bad apples in the bunch, nevertheless the great majority of physicians that we associate with put the care, safety and concerns of our patients first and monetary issues second." They said the article was "disingenuous and counterproductive . . . It would be impossible for our group to support any physician who spouts such self-destructive, one-sided opinions. If this is the opinion of the Department of Cardiology, support of such a department would also become more problematic."

Though I believed in what I had written, I was still nervous. One can never underestimate how hard people will fight to protect their turf. And although my chief was generally supportive of my journalism, I couldn't help thinking of what Santo Russo, my Columbia mentor, had told me in my first year as an attending: "If you mess up relations with a referrer, you can get fired."

One morning, several days after the article was published, Rajiv found me in my office. He closed the door. "No one loves you more than I do," he said, sitting down, "so I have to tell you that you are fucking up." I stared at him but didn't say anything. "You sit in this office all day. You keep the fellows and your patients waiting. I know how smart you are, but you are just so . . . disengaged. And then you write these goddamned articles for the paper! Get it together. People are watching. Don't wait for a crisis to change."

No question, I was in a rut. The strain at home and at work had taken its toll. "You always look so pensive," a colleague told me, and undoubtedly I had, for months. I had accomplished few of the goals I'd set for myself when I started my heart failure program four years earlier. Though I'd helped reduce length of stay and readmissions and had written an admission order set that was being used throughout the hospital, most of my good intentions remained unfulfilled. I knew I couldn't go on like this for much longer. I'd experienced periods of depression before—most recently during internship, when I was exhausted and sleep-deprived for the better part of a year—but this was different, a murkier feeling, as if there were something I was supposed to be worried about but I didn't know what it was, as if I were waiting for something to happen that wasn't happening, so I kept waiting and waiting, sort of hoping it would happen—whatever it was—and be done with.

One day I received an unexpected phone call. Chester Thomas, a young patient of mine, had died suddenly.

Chester was diagnosed with heart failure when he was eighteen years old, but as is so often the case with this disease of manifold etiologies, we never figured out how he got it. He was a student at a community college in Brooklyn when I met him, though he dropped out when his condition worsened. He had short, curly hair and gold wire-framed glasses that rested on the bridge of a wide nose. Despite the setbacks, he was a model patient, coming in diligently with his mother for weekly appointments, eliminating salt from his diet, taking his medications regularly. "May God bless you," his mother often said to me. "You are doing such a wonderful thing for my son. You will be rewarded."

As Chester's condition deteriorated, he started going frequently to the emergency room with abdominal pain. "I was having the dry heaves," he once explained when I admitted him to the hospital. "Sometimes I wonder whether it's psychological. My stomach gets full, the whole abdomen gets hard, like I had nine meals," a result, no doubt, of fluid buildup caused by his weakened heart.

Eventually I referred Chester to a transplant center in Manhattan, where he went for evaluation and frequent follow-up visits. He had to lose weight to qualify for a heart transplant, and by the time he did, his lungs had become so waterlogged that he was suffering from severe fatigue and shortness of breath.

Two weeks before his twentieth birthday, Chester attended a weeklong religious retreat with friends in Kentucky. His doctors, including a transplant cardiologist, had strongly discouraged him from going, but he had insisted. He left by car on a Sunday. The following Friday, he died alone in a hotel room in Lexington.

His mother called to tell me the news. Voice breaking, she thanked John and me for treating him over so many months. She invited us to the funeral.

The church, in Jamaica, Queens, resounded with lilting hymns as we arrived. Inside, men were dressed in cream-colored suits and women in Sunday finery. An organ was playing eerie music in the high-ceilinged chamber. Two men stood in front of the coffin, which carried a portrait of Chester wearing a pinstriped suit, looking debonair, unlike the debilitated state in which I remembered him. As we took our seats, a man in a yellow suit got up and started tap dancing, exhorting the crowd to come up and dance with him. A woman carried a shrieking toddler to the back of the room.

Soon people were clapping on tambourines and playing harmonicas in fast, crazy rhythms. Men came up to praise Chester. "He walked with God . . . He is in a better place . . . He never did nothing the wrong way." One person confirmed what I'd always known about Chester: "He believed in order and had no tolerance for cutting corners." A few folks were dancing wildly as Gospels were shouted. "Speak praise of the Lord," someone bellowed. "You can hear me say it now: the Almighty himself will lead you down the path of the true and the righteous."

Chester's uncle, a bishop, stood up and delivered the main eulogy.

In soaring oratory he declared that Chester had had an unshakable conviction that God would save him. "Even in his worst sickness, when he had to tell his brothers to give him a few minutes because he could not get up from a chair—even then he had faith." The audience roared its approval.

"Ticktock!" he screamed into a microphone, which reverberated in dissonant feedback. "Your time is coming, too. Keep on with the insults, the small-minded bruises and disputes. Ticktock! Your time is coming, too." Murmurings swelled to shouts of support. Someone opened the coffin. Chester lay in repose, his skin gray, his eyes closed. A shiver spread across my chest.

"Ticktock!" Again and again he shouted these words as I sat transfixed, my eyes filling with tears at the spectacle. I thought of my trip to Fargo and all the silly acrimony with my father. What was the point of it when our time together was going to end anyway? How strange this existence, I told myself. It is the finitude of life that keeps us going, and yet it saps meaning from our lives if this is all there is.

The sermon then took on a more subdued tone. The uncle recalled how Chester had been adopted as an infant. (I had not known.) He said Chester had taught himself Hebrew and liked being called T.R., for Temple Rabbi. (Another thing I hadn't known.) Then he said, "Forgive me, but I want to focus on the lighter side of my nephew." He told how Chester enjoyed wearing stylish clothes. He recalled Chester's youthful indiscretions. "Chester loved White Castle cheeseburgers." I did a double take: Cheeseburgers loaded with sodium? Chester had always denied such improprieties to us. "And chicken rolls with soy sauce. Whenever he was with me, we would always stop for takeout."

I looked at John. He had the same disbelieving look I must have had.

"Chester did not like taking his medications," his uncle went on, as if speaking to me. "I'd remind him to do it, force him to, but he would avoid it because they didn't make him feel good." I shifted uncomfortably in my seat. "And you all know he never wanted a heart transplant. He never would have accepted one." (That was news to me, too.)

Afterward, John and I were asked to say a few words. John recalled how much Chester loved pens, how John always gave him a fancy pen when he came to see us. (I'd had no idea.) He said he believed that God had put us on this earth for a reason and that Chester had fulfilled his purpose in this world. Then it was my turn. As I walked up, I thought about the signs I'd missed while taking care of Chester. I thought about how easy it is to ignore social milieu, habits, the sorts of things that make a patient into a real person—and vice versa. Undoubtedly, such information would have helped me treat Chester while he was alive. Standing behind the podium, I told the crowd that Chester was brave and vibrant. I called his death a tragedy. Then I thanked his adoptive mother for inviting me. I had learned so much that day.

After the service, John and I went to a nearby deli for lunch. "There is always someone who has it worse than you," John said after we sat down. "No matter how bad things get."

I nodded and took a bite of my pastrami sandwich. I was hungry.

"People don't take the long view," John went on, uncharacteristically philosophical. "We worry about so much trivial stuff."

I smiled at John's gravity, but he was right, of course. We so often waste our borrowed time. I had seen so much death the past four years, seen so many patients come and go. A few weeks prior, when I had been in line at the hospital deli to buy an iced coffee, a woman in front of me paid for her drink, picked up a laptop computer and a sheaf of papers, and turned to me in my white coat and said, "He's probably dead by now, my husband," and walked out. It had been overwhelming at times— I could never forget the horrible ways by which Joseph Cimino and Lily Dunhill had died—but I had become almost inured to it, and I didn't feel so afraid of it anymore. I often thought of a letter I'd received from the mother of another young patient of mine, a man in his early twenties who'd been born with severe congenital heart defects—a large hole between the upper cardiac chambers, an incompletely formed left ventricle—requiring multiple surgeries. She'd written:

All of life is snatched from death. Our responsibility is to fully taste it. I believe that we each live many lifetimes, that none of us is a stranger to the other. I believe that temporal time, as we perceive it, is an illusion. And so the part of me that is not the grieving mother knows deeply in her heart that the duration of this lifetime of Jack's is not what really matters. And that any attempt to cling to it only ends in despair.

It was impossible, with all the death I had witnessed, not to think about how I was eventually going to die. Was I going to cling to life in desperation? Would death happen suddenly, as for my grandfather? Would it drag out, with me helpless at the epicenter, like Lily Dunhill? Or would I accept it with equanimity like Leonard Sullivan? Sullivan, a patient I took care of for almost three years, loved the sea, loved to sail his little catboat on Long Island Sound. "I must go down to the seas again" is the beginning of "Sea Fever," a poem his son, a college professor, told me he recited countless times, sometimes to express his sense of awe about the sea and sailing ships, sometimes to express his frustration that he was living in a home in suburbia rather than leading the sailor's "vagrant gypsy life." When he entered the terminal phase of his disease, his wife insisted on the most aggressive treatment possible, but Sullivan rejected it. After he died, his son wrote this letter:

> Near the end of his life, when he was no longer responsive, when the "death rattle" began in his breathing, I read "Sea Fever" to him. As soon as I started reading the poem he rose up in bed and started turning his head from side to side and up and down. What I witnessed I will never forget. We had been talking to him for the last several hours but he seemed not to hear us. But I know he heard that poem, something familiar, something from his past, something etched in his memory and dear to his heart. What I believe, what I want to believe and yet, what I do believe, is that hearing this poem took away my father's fear of death, and that this is the reason why, just five minutes after reading him the poem, he passed away. And what I want to believe is that he passed away, beyond the horizon, on a tall sailing ship, listening to the song of the wind, the seagulls crying, amused by a merry yarn from a laughing fellow rover, feeling the kick of the wheel and the shaking of the sails, living at last that vagrant gypsy life for which he longed so intensely his entire life, and finding, at the end of life's long trick, a quiet sleep and a sweet dream.

SIXTEEN

Follow the Money

I am dying from the treatment of too many physicians.

—Alexander the Great

Pia was born on July 1, the date that medical school graduates start their internships. When people ask me if she is "Daddy's girl," I am reminded that human relationships are constrained by biology. Girls so often fancy their fathers. Even my sister, Suneeta: though she spent so little time with my busy father growing up, she still adored him. Dad always says how wonderful it is to have a daughter. Girls are more sincere, he says. And loyal.

Our baby girl and her accoutrements quickly swallowed up the little remaining space in our apartment. We put her crib in Mohan's room and had him sleep with us, throwing off his schedule, which started to conform more and more to ours. It was a subpar solution, but there was little else we could do. The hourglass had turned, and Sonia and I both knew our time in Manhattan was coming to an end.

The prospect of suburban living created a peculiar polarity in my mind. I feared the loneliness and insularity of the suburbs—was there anything more depressing than the manicured patch of lawn in front of the local bank?—and yet my remembrances of my suburban upbringing were mostly fond ones. (Or had I just filtered away the terribleness?) I'd grown up in Southern California, at the edge of the desert—a wasteland, and not just because of the cacti—and though I now fancied myself an urban guy, I had vaguely happy memories of my childhood: dirt biking on the dunes behind the train tracks, catching crickets in the backyard at dusk, playing touch football on the street at night, scuffing my knees on the gray asphalt.

Of course, it was a very different time from today. There was little parental supervision; mothers and fathers didn't feel compelled to be their kids' best friends or social secretaries. Nowadays there is such little tolerance for ignorance about our children's whereabouts, but back then, at least in our middle-class neighborhood, it was the norm. Most of the moms had full-time jobs. My friend Billy's dad worked nights at the printing press, so though he stayed at home during the day to supervise, he slept most of the time—he was morbidly obese and had sleep apnea to boot—and we were left largely to our own imaginations. We'd thumb through Stevie's dad's collection of *Playboys* and *Penthouses*. We'd ogle our friend Sammy's older sister, Jessica, sunbathing topless (or so we wanted to believe), through a hole in the fence. We scaled a hundred feet up the exterior of the clock tower at the local university. Once, we even considered jumping off Billy's roof into his swimming pool, desisting only after Carl, a kid from up the street, deemed it a bad idea. But moving out of the city wasn't about nostalgia or reliving a lost time or providing a more natural place for my children to grow up. It was essentially about a lack of space, and the lack of money to buy more.

———

Because insurers had been slashing reimbursement rates, that summer my LIJ colleagues and I were told we had to increase our "relative value unit" collections, or RVUs (the currency of medical payment). With all the cuts in reimbursements over the prior few years, academic medical departments across the country had suffered sharp downturns in revenue. Some physicians had responded by upcoding—claiming greater complexity in patient encounters than was in fact the case—and fraud investigations at some centers were under way. Obviously I wasn't going to upcode, so what the department's directive meant for me on a practical level was that I had to see more patients. I reduced the time in my schedule earmarked for new patients from sixty minutes to forty and for established patients from thirty minutes to twenty. With administrative tasks, conferences, teaching, chart reviews, and letters and phone calls to physicians, hospitals, and pharmacies increasingly gobbling up my day, I began to rush through visits, hurrying patients along in subtle and not so subtle ways. I stopped making small talk. I interrupted histories after a few seconds to get patients on point. I even urged my patients to breathe a little faster when I was listening to their lungs. "Doctor, I just want to know . . ." "One second, ma'am, please, one second . . ."

With the added density in my schedule, I started to cut corners. I discovered that one of my patients had herpes zoster—shingles—which would have fully explained her chest pains. The ER didn't pick up on it, and neither did I or two cardiology fellows who examined her. She noticed the telltale rash only while she was bathing, after undergoing a costly and unnecessary cardiac workup. "It's pathetic," I wrote in my journal. "We don't open our eyes, and what did I do with the next patient? I still didn't disrobe him to examine him properly. I can't believe I've become like this. I hate myself for not trying harder."

You can often do a passable job, but it is impossible to appreciate the subtleties of patient care when you are rushing. Kenneth Ludmerer, a physician and medical historian at Washington University in St. Louis, has said that "the single greatest problem in medicine today is the disrespect of time. One cannot do anything in medicine well on the fly." So, racing through patient encounters, you practice with an ever-present fear that you will miss something, hurt someone, and open yourself up to legal (not to mention moral) liability. To cope with the anxiety, you start to call in "experts" for problems that perhaps you could have handled yourself if you had had more time to think through the case. Apart from the perverse incentives of our fee-for-service system, a major driver of overconsultation is the uncertainty engendered by the hurried pace of contemporary medicine. Some doctors call consults just to "cover their ass." Sometimes the "easy" consults are the hardest ones, not because you don't know what to do but because you have to figure out why you were called in the first place. Wanton consultation is a consequence of the zip drive of modern medicine, in which patients are compressed into a smaller and smaller space-time.

One of my patients, Nora Mitchell, went to the ER after swallowing a tiny fishbone. She told me about the experience when she came to see me. "They kept me down in that ER for two days, Dr. Jauhar!

They did X-rays, EKGs, CT scans, God knows what. They had an ENT doctor come by. They called a pulmonologist. They told me to follow up with my cardiologist. I told them it had nothing to do with it. It was the fish!"

The Institute of Medicine, a respected think tank, recently estimated that wasteful health care spending—spending that does not improve health outcomes—costs $750 billion in the United States every year. Excessive paperwork and administrative costs explain some of this waste, but unnecessary or inefficiently delivered services, especially in hospitals, account for the lion's share.

This is the sad irony of the cost containment paradigm. The more pressure on doctors to cut costs by working harder and faster, with shorter hospital stays and quicker patient turnover, the more uncertainty doctors often feel, and therefore the more likely they are to utilize CT scans, MRIs, expert consultations, and so on. There is no more wasteful entity in medicine than a rushed (or incompetent) doctor.

The consequences for patients are troubling. Having too many consultants leads to sloppiness and disorganization. Mr. Wolski complained about this when I went to his hospital room one morning. "Man, there are really some incompetents in this place. Around midnight, I'm eating something and a nurse comes by and says, 'Nothing by mouth after midnight.' After midnight, some character comes upstairs and says, 'I think you're going for dialysis.' I asked him, 'How do you know? Am I or not?' but he didn't have a clue. He said he'd check, but he never came back. This morning, in comes Dr. Richards. He was amazed that no one had dropped a central catheter in me, so they did that." He shook his head in disgust. "Then it turns out no one did blood tests and they needed to find out what my Coumadin level was, so they ran around doing that. Then they came in at eleven-thirty this morning and cheerfully said, 'You're going to dialysis.' They took me downstairs. I started feeling sick. I asked them to let me dangle my legs over the side of the stretcher, but they wouldn't let me. I couldn't get it through to them. Nobody listened!"

With bulky care teams, there is diffusion of responsibility. Who's in charge? Who is spearheading treatment? Nowhere is this confusion more evident than in the hospital discharge process.

In 2009 a study in *The New England Journal of Medicine* found that one in five Medicare patients discharged from the hospital was readmitted within a month. One in three was readmitted within three months. Readmissions, so plentiful, are costly. In 2004 the expense to Medicare for unplanned readmissions was $17.4 billion—17 percent of its total hospital budget.

Hasty readmission is an indicator of an inefficient, if not dysfunctional, health care system. Many factors contribute to the problem: poor communication, inadequate discharge instructions, spotty information transfer, and delayed outpatient follow-up. And all these things derive in part from the lack of time health care providers have for patients.

Doctors working in hospitals are increasingly rushed. The arsenal of tests, therapies, and technologies is more complex. Resident work schedules have less total and consecutive hours, so there are more handoffs and less continuity of care and attending physicians have had to take on more responsibilities than in the past. As Dr. Donald Berwick and Dr. Allan Detsky recently wrote in *The Journal of the American Medical Association*, inpatient care at teaching hospitals has become a relay race for physicians and consultants, and patients are the batons. In a recent study of nearly three thousand adults, 75 percent of inpatients were unable to name a single doctor assigned to their care. Of the remaining quarter who offered a name, 60 percent were wrong.

There are many things doctors could do to reduce hospital readmission rates. They could ensure that discharged patients get timely followup appointments. (In the *New England Journal* study, half of all medical patients readmitted within thirty days had not visited a doctor after discharge.) They could do a better job of ensuring that patients obtained their medications and understood how to take them. When I was a fellow, one of my elderly patients bounced back to the hospital simply because she'd missed her morning dose of diuretic on the day after discharge. Though I'd given her prescriptions and gone over the dosing schedule, I hadn't checked whether there was someone available to drive to the pharmacy to get her medications, an oversight that resulted in a $10,000 rehospitalization. Doctors could also do a better job of educating patients about which symptoms and signs presage worsening of their disease—shortness of breath and leg swelling in congestive heart failure, for example—so they could quickly see their primary physicians rather than go to the emergency room. We know that patients with a clear understanding of discharge instructions are 30 percent less likely to return to the hospital. But research shows inconsistency at best in achieving these goals.

After so many years in medicine, I am convinced of one thing: The vast majority of doctors aren't bad. It is the system that makes us bad, makes us make mistakes. Most doctors—and this is certainly true of my colleagues at the hospital—are willing to stay late and work hard to provide good care. But they are struggling to do so in a system that is diseased. I often think of Dr. Nelson from my residency days at New York Presbyterian Hospital. A retired old-timer, he'd come to all our morning reports. He'd hold special teaching rounds with the residents. We'd groan when he came around because we didn't have the time to spend an hour on one patient. But he showed us the ideal, how best to approach a difficult case, even if you could reach it only every once in a while. Still, people used to whisper about Nelson. He'd had a busy practice. He used to be a terror with residents, dismissive of his patients. So over time he obviously had to change, too.

To curb health costs, Congress and the Obama administration are now doling out penalties (as of October 1, 2012) on hospitals with high readmission rates. Hospitals, many with very narrow margins, could forfeit up to 1 percent of Medicare payments in 2013, 2 percent in 2014, and 3 percent in 2015 and after. But these incentives are misdirected. Hospitals do not hospitalize patients; doctors do. And doctors currently stand to gain little from lowering readmissions. In fact, they will lose revenue. As is so often the case in our health care system, doctors' incentives do not serve broader social goals. This virtually guarantees that proposed reforms like cutting readmissions, reducing unnecessary testing, and adopting computerized medical records will fail.

The agency that runs Medicare is considering giving bonuses to hospitals that lower readmissions below the average. Though I think it's a good idea, I believe some of this money should be shared with doctors. Current law prohibits hospitals from paying doctors for reducing hospital services, even if the goal is to provide more efficient care. But such "gainsharing" will align physicians' incentives with cost-cutting goals. Our system, structured to encourage overutilization, needs to provide some inducements to reduce the amount of health care, too.

You have to motivate doctors to do the right thing. You can appeal to professionalism or altruism, to doing well for patients or serving a greater social purpose, but as I have come to learn, nothing today influences physicians' behavior (even if unconsciously) like hard cash. If you want to understand why doctors behave the way they do, look at the schedule of Medicare payments. As in politics, just follow the money.

SEVENTEEN

Speed Dating

We trust our health to the physician . . . Their reward must be such, therefore, as may give them that rank in the society which so important a trust requires.   —Adam Smith, *The Wealth of Nations*, 1776

Despite the increased workload at the hospital, I needed to find another moonlighting opportunity to make up for the shortfall in income. Though I knew I'd have to purchase my own malpractice policy, I figured it would be worthwhile if I earned at least $35,000 per year moonlighting, roughly double the insurance premium. But notwithstanding searching for several months, I was unable to find a regular gig like the one I'd had with Chaudhry. An imaging company was looking for a cardiologist to supervise its New York City operations. "You can expect a contract to arrive in your hands in the first part of September," a sales rep promised me in an e-mail, adding that I could make roughly $700 per week, but I never heard from him again. A private cardiologist told me that an outfit in Queens called Daval Diagnostics was looking for someone to read its nuclear stress tests, but when she called on my behalf, the manager wanted to know if I'd be referring my own patients for testing. "They want to know what you can bring to the table," she explained. So that fell through, too.

Since I was taking doc-of-the-day calls every week, I reached out to private internists who had clinical privileges at the hospital, offering them "general medical consults" on my ER patients, wishfully thinking that if I built up my referral network, Chaudhry might take me back. It was a different sort of challenge: beating a flawed system, finding a way to extract what I needed. Though mercenary, it still held a peculiar kind of attraction.

However, my efforts fizzled badly. Most internists I contacted weren't interested in coming to the hospital. One of them straight-out told me not to call him; he was trying to eliminate his inpatient work. (Later I discovered he was doing the same consults for another cardiologist.) It was embarrassing, really, trying to practice quid pro quo medicine— and failing. Perhaps the internists found me ingratiating or my designs too obvious. Perhaps referral patterns were already set. Perhaps my efforts weren't backed up by jocularity or friendship. Or maybe I just wasn't the kind of person who could pull it off.

At Rajiv's urging, I invited his friend Sameer Chawla, the private internist Chaudhry and I had once courted, out to dinner. The three of us met one muggy summer evening at an Indian restaurant near the hospital. Sameer was a short man, faintly canine, with a knotted beard and a small bhag turban. The evening started off well. Rajiv ordered Black Label Scotch and a platter of lamb chops, Punjabi style, the Rajiv Jauhar appetizer special ("I come here so much, they named a dish after me!"). We gossiped about medicine on Long Island: private practices being bought up by hospitals, Medicare fraud audits, and so on. Sameer told us about nursing home doctors who hospitalized patients with false diagnoses like "altered mental status," admitting these patients through a network of colluding physicians so monitors wouldn't detect the deceit. He mentioned pharmacists in Queens who were offering physicians bribes for fake prescriptions that the pharmacists would then submit to insurers for reimbursement. "Imagine getting one hundred percent profit from Medicaid!" he exclaimed. I listened in disbelief.

Midway through bowls of spicy chicken makhani and saag paneer, I gently brought up the subject of referrals. Rajiv had advised me to tell Sameer that I was still partnered with Chaudhry and that we were trying to generate more business. So I suggested the following arrangement: Chaudhry and I would rent space in Sameer's office, Sameer would provide us patients, and all resulting cardiac procedures would be done back at Chaudhry's workplace. But Sameer immediately dismissed the idea, saying he didn't want anyone coming to his office. When he left to go to the bathroom, Rajiv shrugged and said, "He does things by the book," of course making me feel even worse. It was bad enough trying to make a backroom deal, but I couldn't even get *that* done. When Sameer returned, he asked me about Sonia. I told him that she had just passed her internal medicine board exams but was at home for the time being, taking care of our newborn. He encouraged me to move to Long Island. "Put your wife to work," he said. "We will keep her busy." I told him I'd mention it to Sonia.

I didn't want to take another handout from Sonia's father, so in desperation I again reached out to Chaudhry's associate Malik to help me find additional work. At first he counseled caution—"you don't want to get involved with doctors you don't know"—but eventually he relented and suggested a few practices. So for a couple of months I found myself zipping around Queens and Long Island after my regular workday, rushing to make six o'clock meetings with internists or owners of testing facilities looking for someone to do their cardiac work. Malik's friend Rakesh, a former stress test technician at NYU who was trying to build a business as a nuclear isotope supplier, frequently accompanied me to these conferences. Rakesh was a wiry Indian with a nervous smile and an unfortunately severe stammer. He once took me to meet a Malaysian businessman who called himself Johnny Miller. The meeting was to take place in a sterile office building in Jericho, New York, called (appropriately enough) the Atrium. We arrived a bit early.

"He wants to open up f-f-full-service cardiac centers with consultation and imaging," Rakesh told me while we sat at a Starbucks next door, plotting my strategy. "He'll s-s-say a lot of things, d-drop a lot of names. I don't know whether he's knowing these people or not. Best to say as l-little as possible. Don't say two words when one will do."

"He sounds like a crook," I said, already regretting that I had agreed to come.

Rakesh started laughing. "You try to G-Google him, and nothing comes up, no trace of him or his company, yet he claims to run a multimillion-dollar business. I don't know if he's hiding his money or using a false name or whatnot, but that is none of your c-c-concern."

"I'm not sure this is going to be such a good fit," I said nervously. Just being at that strip mall felt shady, illicit—and sort of titillating, too.

"Just s-see what he has to say. Make it w-w-work for you."

Inside the building we took an elevator to the second floor. The wood-paneled hallway was carpeted in vomit beige. A woman came out to greet us and took us into a conference room, where we sat at a table and waited.

Before long, Mr. Miller came in. He was a jowly, dark-skinned fellow with shiny white teeth and a sort of affected nonchalance. He started off by making strange small talk, asking me personal questions, the origins of my name, whether it was Muslim, and so on.

"I grew up in Kuala Lumpur," he said. "There were many Muslims."

"No, no, he is H-Hindu," Rakesh assured him, as I looked on awkwardly. "He is from Punjab. Some went to P-P-Pakistan in the Partition. Some stayed in India." Mr. Miller immediately appeared more at ease.

He eventually got around to telling me that he wanted to create full-service diagnostic centers where doctors not only would do procedures but would evaluate and manage patients, too. "Otherwise you have to keep feeding the primary care physicians for referrals," he explained. "Then we are no better than Daval Diagnostics." He told me that he already had a cardiologist on the payroll but that he needed to find a replacement because that doctor wasn't board-certified. "He's not proud of it. He's studying for the board exams now. But there you go," he said with a dismissive flick of the hand. More and more insurers, Miller explained, were refusing to pay for echos and stress tests ordered by non-board-certified cardiologists. "The last two patients we saw, we couldn't bill for any noninvasive testing. One patient had asthma with coronary risk factors. You should do an echo, right?" Before I could respond, he said, "But we couldn't do it. There's no point doing the studies if we are not going to get paid."

He had previously worked with a doctor who had been billing tests with his own provider number (something I didn't quite understand), so all reimbursement checks had gone to him rather than to Miller. That doctor had left Miller high and dry. Miller said he was owed over $30,000. So that relationship had been a disaster, too.

"For echo, we get about three hundred dollars," he went on. "For nukes, about six hundred and fifty. You can still make money on nukes, but I have to pay the technician, buy the isotope, cover the lease fee." He was muttering numbers—"twelve thousand, sixteen thousand"—computing in his head. Finally he said, "So I am prepared to pay you forty dollars per echo and fifty-five for a nuclear reading. But the rest of

the insurance money has to get paid to us in the form of rent. Fee split-
ting is illegal, and I don't want to do anything illegal. The last thing I
need is to get anyone else on my ass."

He asked me when I wanted to get started. I told him I'd get back
to him.

A few weeks later, Rakesh told me that Mr. Miller had disappeared.
Rakesh had left several voice messages that had not been returned. "It's
a b-b-bad situation," he said nervously. "B-b-best not to g-g-go there."

Of course, I felt disgusted with myself. Four years earlier I'd decided
to specialize in congestive heart failure because I wanted to develop
long-term relationships with patients. I'd made what I considered a moral
choice; income wasn't part of the calculation. Now everything had been
turned upside down. The words of Dr. Dowton, my medical school
commencement speaker, often flashed through my mind: "Work out
what things in life you care about, the beliefs you hold near and dear,
and stick to them." I'd been so busy trying to navigate the new world in
which I had landed that I hadn't given much thought to this advice.
The past four years at LIJ had been such a turbulent time, both professionally and personally. I'd been so occupied with the heavy lifting of
establishing my career that I hadn't given much thought to my "value
system" or to the kind of doctor—and I don't mean specialist—that I
wanted to be.

But now, as I was skirting the murky border into knavery, a decision
was at hand. When I stepped back and looked at what I'd been doing for
nearly two years, I almost couldn't believe that I was the same person
who had decided to become a heart failure specialist. I had been buoyed
by the force of a nebulous idea: that it wasn't really I who had subverted
the ideals with which I'd entered my profession—giving paid talks for
pharmaceutical companies, working with someone like Chaudhry—but
some other person being forced by circumstance. However, this ratio-
nalization was starting to break down. I was rapidly approaching the
point where I had to make another moral choice.

Malik knew an internist named Anwar Hasani on the South Shore
of Long Island who was doing very well—making close to a million dollars a year, Malik claimed—and needed a cardiologist to read his studies. "How is it he's making more than five times what an average primary
care doctor makes?" I asked. "Is it just about procedures?"

"Of course it's about procedures," Malik replied, "but how do you get procedures? Some guys have no clue how to do it. I told one doctor I was working for, this patient can get a thyroid sonogram, this one a kidney ultrasound, that one a nerve conduction study, peripheral vascular, carotid, echo, stress echo, but he had no clue how to make it happen. Guys like Amir and Hasani treat it as a business. Do the study as long as it isn't illegal. The patients don't mind."

By then I had seen enough of the underbelly of private practice to be unfazed by such a sordid remark. "Who reads his studies now?" I asked.

"Some guy named Ferraro. But they had a falling-out. He is looking to make a change."

Malik took me to see Hasani one evening after work. We parked next door in the lot of an electronics emporium. "Don't tell Amir I came with you," Malik said, furtively checking the rearview mirror. "He hates Hasani."

"Why?"

"He used to read Hasani's studies, but Hasani never paid him. He owes him a lot of money."

Wearily, I opened the car door. I could hardly believe I was spending another evening away from my family.

"Hasani wants to do more carotid ultrasounds," Malik said.

"I don't read carotids," I said immediately.

"Well, hear what he has to say. He has a lot of volume. He could open a lot of doors for you."

"Honestly, I don't know if I'm going to have the time," I said, just wanting to go home.

"If you spread it on the table, it won't be as much work as you think," Malik said encouragingly. I stepped out of the car. "Just remember, he is a businessman," Malik said in parting. "He is going to lowball you. That's why he drives a Bentley."

Hasani kept me waiting in his cramped office for half an hour while he discussed something with his office manager. (Malik remained in the parking lot.) When Hasani finally walked in, I was feeling unusually edgy. I had just scratched a scab off my shin. Blood was trickling down my leg as I swabbed the wound with my bare, reddened fingertips. Unperturbed, he handed me a box of tissues.

He was in his mid-fifties, a short, balding Egyptian with a stethoscope draped over a fashionable beige turtleneck. He sat down in a red leather chair behind his desk. He spoke slowly and deliberately, with the confidence of the owner of a successful enterprise.

"The most important thing is that we have good studies," he said once we started discussing the work arrangement. "I will give you a tape and you tell me if it meets your standards."

I nodded, wanting to get out of there.

"I want only one person, so you'll have to read carotid ultrasounds, too," he said. (That meant interpreting digital images he'd provide on a compact disc.)

"Well, as I explained on the phone, I am not yet certified in carotids."

"That's okay," he said quickly. "The insurance companies are not requiring board certification at this time anyway. I suggest you get trained quickly, but meanwhile, you should just start reading. Most of the studies are normal anyway. If anyone has real pathology, I send them to the hospital to repeat the test."

I must have squirmed, but I didn't say anything.

"We don't want a rental arrangement," Hasani continued. "We want to do the billing ourselves. I want you to run my whole cardiovascular program: reading echos, supervising echos, doing consultations and stress tests. If you can take over my entire service, you can make eight thousand dollars a month. Once we start nuclears, you can make an extra fifteen hundred to two thousand a month." He wanted me to help him accredit his echo and stress labs, too. In short, he said, he was looking for a "comprehensive arrangement."

I told him I would think it over and discuss it with my department head.

"We want your hospital name on the building," he said quickly. "We are talking to St. Francis and Winthrop, too. But if your hospital is looking to do the billing and just pay me rent, then it won't work out."

When I got back to the parking lot, Malik was still waiting in the car. "So what do you think?" he said.

I replied that I didn't think the hospital would agree to Hasani's terms.

"Well, see what they say," he said, starting the car. "Everybody is trying to make money. That's the bottom line."

As Malik drove back to Queens, chattering about this and that, I remained lost in thought, paying only intermittent attention. I ran my fingers across my sweaty brow. *You have to get out of this situation and never come back*, I told myself. *You don't want to feel this way anymore. It's not about anyone else. It's about you, who you are and what you do, how you receive the gifts that are your life.*

At one point, Malik mentioned that Hasani had applied for a state inspection to start a nuclear lab. "A nuclear is serious stuff," Malik said. "I asked him, 'Do you know who's going to stand in front of this thing and going to monitor this stuff?' and he said, 'Oh, I haven't thought about that yet.' That's how much thought he's put into it."

"Sounds like it's all about the business," I said, gazing absentmindedly out the window.

"Yeah, like a lot of doctors, Hasani just cares about the numbers. Patients come down to the treadmill with a cane. I say, 'Why is this person here for a stress test?' It's like, who's ordering this?"

"Who is ordering it?"

"Him and his PA. I mean, seventy-five-year-old, four stents, diabetic, and I ask why they are having a stress echo. I mean, nuke them if you have to. But he's just biding his time, waiting for his nuclear license."

"He sounds like a dick."

"You're right. Do you know what the litmus test is? Amir could not work with him. And Amir would sell his mother for a few more dollars. If Amir couldn't work with Hasani, that should tell you something."

I stared at the road ahead. This was not how things were supposed to have turned out. At the very least, this was not the conception of doctoring that I'd had when I started in practice. Of course, you're supposed to make compromises as you get older, as you accrue responsibilities for other people—your children, your spouse, your parents—but it felt as if I had made a Faustian bargain. Having my eyes opened to the reality of contemporary medical practice had been painful. Now I had to make a choice. Continuing on this path was leading to ruin.

"We are in a terrible situation as doctors," Malik said. "Things are drying up. Before, when you mentioned diabetes—boom!—you got approved. Now you say even chest pain and the insurance company has twenty more questions. If the PA ordering the test doesn't know his clinicals, it isn't going to get approved."

By then I had stopped paying attention. What Malik was saying no longer mattered. I wasn't going to work with Hasani or Miller or Fibak or Bennett or anyone else he had introduced me to. I was done driving around, rushing to this place and that, meeting knaves looking to exploit the system, and constantly thinking about how to make more money for myself so we could maintain a life that was probably unsustainable anyway. Just as condensation droplets on a windowpane merge to make a tiny stream, my thoughts at that moment seemed to coalesce. I wasn't going to waste any more time. The way forward had become clear.

EIGHTEEN

Diversion

Childhood's joy-land.
Mystic merry Toyland,
Once you pass its borders,
You can never return again.
—Victor Herbert and Glen MacDonough

The moment when I finally decided it was time to leave Manhattan, I was sprinting across the West Side Highway through heavy traffic. It was a bright Saturday afternoon in the summer, five years after I'd started working at LIJ. That morning, Matt, a lawyer who lived in my building, had invited me to play tennis at 119th Street in Riverside Park, but since our passes had expired, we weren't allowed to get on a court. Someone told us you didn't need a pass to play on the red clay courts at 96th Street, so we decided to walk there. It was a beautiful day. Sailboats were out on the shimmering Hudson, and fluffy white clouds extended like a mattress across the light blue sky. When we arrived, forty minutes later, all the courts were occupied, and because we didn't have valid passes, we weren't allowed to reserve a court for later in the afternoon. If we were willing to wait, a court might open up, but it was impossible to predict when that would happen. Someone told us there were public courts at the middle school on 116th Street and Lenox, so, desperate to play, we decided to walk back uptown.

The bridge over the West Side Highway was at 125th Street, and because we didn't want to waste time walking an extra eighteen blocks, we impulsively decided to cross the highway right where we were. Cars whizzed by us as we took refuge between lanes, as if we were participating in a real-life game of Frogger. It was at that moment, risking my life for a chance to play tennis, that I decided I no longer wanted to live in Manhattan. Even if I were to find more moonlighting work, the sacrifices required were just too great. Sonia, frantically trying to enroll in overcrowded "Mommy and me" classes, had begun to feel the same way. (And the courts at the school turned out to be unplayable anyway.)

In the fall, we started to look in earnest for a house. It wasn't a perfect solution to our financial situation, but at least it would allow me to forgo any more private moonlighting. I had convinced Sonia that I couldn't make the commute daily from New Jersey, so almost every weekend, Sonia, Mohan, and I (we left Pia at home with a babysitter) drove out to Long Island and walked the naked floors of homes for sale in Manhasset and Roslyn. We looked at single-family houses, rentals, condos, even gated communities, but nothing seemed quite right. The centrifugal force of our financial troubles was balanced by the competing weights of inertia and familiarity. I tried to picture us in a suburban house, easily putting our well-rested kids in their cute animal pajamas to bed and then retiring to a den with a fireplace, an armchair, and high bookshelves, but it was all so hard to imagine. What was I going to do at night without the buzz from the street to soothe me to sleep? When Sonia asked me what was wrong, I told her I was worried about Mohan, about taking him away from his school, his friends, his neighborhood— were we being fair to him, changing his way of life?—but in truth I was more worried about myself.

With generous help from my father-in-law, we eventually signed a contract of sale for a three-bedroom house in the town of Glen Head, about a fifteen-minute drive from LIJ. By then, Mohan had a vague idea that we were moving, though I'd never sat down to talk with him about it. I dreaded telling him.

Shortly after the purchase was finalized, I took my son for our usual Saturday outing in Riverside Park. He looked adorable in his Bermuda shorts and green polo shirt. At the corner of 110th and Broadway, we negotiated where to go first.

"I want to go to the park," he said.

"Let's first go to the bookstore," I said.

"No, park."

"Come on, can we go to the bookstore for a minute?"

He thought for a moment. Then, like an old friend, he said, "You want to see your book?" (The paperback had been released.)

At the bookstore, he sat quietly while I perused the new titles. He whispered to himself as I thumbed through periodicals. Then we sat in a chair, and I read him *Little Quack*, about ducklings reluctant to move to a different pond. When we were done, we rode the escalator back upstairs. He mimicked my stance, straddling two steps with his diminutive legs. Outside on the sidewalk, he cried out in relief: "We can talk now! We can talk now! We can be loud now! I'm so happy!"

Since we were already at 115th Street, we cut through the Columbia campus. Mohan sprinted in front of me. On the main plaza he dunked his hands into the brackish fountain, breaking through the muck of feathers and cigarette butts floating on the surface. I asked him if he wanted to climb to the top of the stairs and watch people—my favorite pastime at Berkeley—but he wanted to run. So we ran around on the grass in front of the math library, trying to scare squirrels.

I'd been promising to take him to the dinosaur playground, so we walked down to the subway to catch a train going downtown. When we got out at Ninety-sixth Street, throngs were out on the sidewalk. I carried Mohan through the crowd. Music was blaring, and street vendors were peddling their wares. "So many scooters and bicycles and motorcycles," Mohan cried. "It's such a beautiful day!"

On the way to the playground, we walked by his school. "Mr. Tabakin doesn't like James," he said.

"Why?" I asked.

"Because James eats candy. Ms. Morrison and Mr. Tabakin said you can't bring candy to school. Not because everybody wants some—that's not the problem—but because it will get disappeared. That means it's gone. That's the problem."

I chuckled. "Mama said James pushed you the other day."

"Yes, he pushed me."

"What did you say to him?"

"I said, 'Don't push me.'"

"And what did he say?"

"He said, 'Okay, I won't push you.'" He smiled, obviously proud of this victory.

By the time we got to the river, he was tired, so I carried him for a ways. Off in the distance, the George Washington Bridge unfurled over the Hudson like a steel bracelet. When we reached the playground, he wiggled out of my arms. "Let's run!" he commanded. I followed him. Almost immediately he was running up the steps of a slide. He glided down the corkscrew and then quickly followed a kid back up to the top to maximize the chance of barreling into him at the bottom.

"Be careful, I don't want you to get hurt," I called out.

"We can fix the hurt, Dadda," he said, before quickly climbing up the steps to give it another go. "We can fix the hurt."

At the other side of the playground we found a girl, about twelve years old, playing with her little brother. At first the little boy and Mohan regarded each other warily, like dogs sniffing out danger. Mohan started doing a sort of dance, his arms moving back and forth in stiff karate-like movements, as if he were weaving a spell. It was an invitation to play. The boy looked on silently, a bit enticed, perhaps even a bit fearful. I quietly watched this act of charm and seduction. Soon they were playing like old friends.

I often think of my own childhood growing up in New Delhi and then California. My playmates and I used to compete in marbles. Those purple alleys and red opals: Hold them up to the light and they'd shimmer. Flick one with your thumb and hit your friend's and you could keep it. Sometimes the marble would lightly graze in the collision. Other times you'd get a clean hit and your marble, imparting its entire momentum, would stop in its tracks, taking the place of the other.

We used to play tops, too. You'd spin your top in the dirt and drag it with a string to try to hit your opponent's top. Whoever's top twirled the longest got a chance to gouge his opponent's with the metal nail at the apex of his own. Nothing was more satisfying than splintering your opponent's top with a short, clean stab.

As boys, we loved measured violence. In California, where my family moved when I was ten, we played pencils. Your opponent would hold his pencil firmly at both ends, and then you'd whack it with the metal tip of your own, bending your pencil with your thumb to get maximal force. If you snapped quick and hard, the other pencil would crack.

Once, I snapped Tony Hernandez's brand-new Ticonderoga. Tony played tackle football. He was the biggest kid in sixth grade. Insulted, he challenged me to a fight after school. It took place on an elevated patch of grass next to the playground. Every boy in the class showed up. I'm not sure why I did. Perhaps out of fear of further offending Tony.

So there was Tony, towering over me, the scrawny immigrant kid with spectacles. I could smell his warm milk breath on my face. Everyone was watching, waiting for someone to make the first move. He circled me silently for what seemed like minutes. Finally, emboldened by the gallery's calls for some action, I cried, "Get off!" and pushed Tony hard in the chest. I don't know why I did it. I was petrified. He could have kicked my ass with one hand tied behind his back, but he backed down. He warned me not to cheat at pencils again and walked away. The other kids left, too, disappointed, I'm sure. I remained at the playground, sobbing out of relief—and perhaps remorse, too, for making Tony lose face.

At the water fountain, Mohan and his new playmate took mouthfuls of water and spit them at each other. Pretty soon we were all running through the sprinklers. After a while we all took some rest on a bench. "How old are you?" the boy asked Mohan.

"I'm five," Mohan replied.

"I'm five, too," the boy said. "My sister is twelve." He asked Mohan how old I was.

"Forty," I replied.

"Forty!" Mohan cried. "Come on, Dadda. That's not a number!"

"Forty is too a number!"

He looked at me sadly. "Oh, that's too bad, Dadda."

There was a thunderclap. I quickly turned. A huge branch of a Dutch elm had come crashing down onto the gray asphalt a few feet from where the children had been standing. It was ten feet long, about a foot in circumference. It would have crushed anyone standing under it. The boys ran over excitedly to inspect the splintery mess. I stared at it in shock. A woman said she was calling 311.

I quickly gathered up our things, and we boarded a bus going back uptown. It sped up Riverside Drive, past busy playgrounds and Parisian-style apartment houses garnished with metal scaffolding. Back in our neighborhood, I picked Mohan up again. The sidewalks were buzzing with the usual Saturday-afternoon mercantile swarm. I asked him if he wanted to go to the diner for lunch. He nodded yes.

A man was playing the trumpet on the sidewalk in front of the restaurant. We went inside and got seated in a booth. I ordered chicken fingers and a strawberry milk shake for Mohan and a cheeseburger and French fries for myself. When the food came, we dug in. Licking his fingers, Mohan said, "This is fun, Dadda. Let's do this every week."

A sad feeling washed over me, as I knew our outings to Riverside Park were coming to an end. We ate in silence. I finally broached the dreaded subject. "Do you want to live in a house with a backyard?"

"Yes," he said, munching on a French fry.

"But it means we have to leave New York."

"Will there be chicken fingers there?"

"Yes, of course, but they'll be from a different place." He looked at me carefully but didn't say anything. "We can still come back and visit James," I said. He remained quiet. A minute passed.

"You'll go to a great new school with a big playground. You'll make new friends."

He nodded, seeming uninterested. I started to say something, but he interrupted me. "I don't want to talk about this anymore," he said.

"Why?" I asked.

"Because I'm tired," he said.

NINETEEN

A Country Husband

One by one, as they march, our comrades vanish from our sight. Be it ours to shed sunshine on their path, to lighten their sorrows by the balm of sympathy, to give them the pure joy of a never-tiring affection.

—Bertrand Russell

The old man was lying on a double bed, on gray sheets that looked as if they needed washing. The sparsely furnished room was permeated with the stuffy smell of sickness and sleep. A tray of food sat untouched on a bedside table. His cheeks were sunken; his skin was the color of stone. His bare legs had a bluish tinge.

We'd been taking care of Hyman Gesselman for almost two years, but because of progressive heart failure, he was no longer able to come to the office to see us. A few weeks back we had started him on a continuous infusion of dobutamine at home to support his failing heart, just as I had done for Joseph Cimino in the hospital three years prior. Gesselman lived on a quiet street about a mile from the hospital. It was fall. The ground was damp, and the tiny lawn in front of the house was already brown and bare. His wife, Elsa, met John and me at the front door and showed us to their bedroom. She was in her early sixties, about fifteen years younger than he was, with cellophane gray hair and masculine worker hands. An émigré from Russia, she had been a health aide to Gesselman's first wife, who had died two years before. He had married Elsa to secure her a green card and permanent residency. Theirs was a fraught relationship. At office visits she would constantly interrupt him, disputing almost everything he said: whether he had slept, whether he had eaten, whether he had tripped or fainted before falling. Vexed, he'd glare at her and say, "I thought we discussed you weren't going to say anything," but there was little he could do to prevent her from speaking her mind.

In the bedroom, he extended his hand to me weakly. I held it for a few seconds. Spidery blue veins zigzagged under the paper-thin, almost translucent skin. I asked him how he was feeling. He nodded vacantly. I checked his pulse, weak but regular, and his jugular veins, which were reedy and congested. I listened to his chest with my stethoscope. He was wheezing, front and back. I checked on the drug infusion settings: 2.5 micrograms per kilogram per minute, as ordered. I surveyed the room: no obvious tripping hazards. I opened the window blinds. As I was getting ready to leave, he stopped me. "My life was travel, Dr. Jauhar," he mumbled. "Arizona, Bar Harbor—will I ever be able to do that again?"

I didn't know how to respond. I knew he would likely never make it out of his house again, let alone travel by plane, but I didn't want to take away all hope. "I don't know, Hyman," I said softly. "Let's see how things go."

Glassy-eyed, he rasped, "I just want to be able to walk. It's so depressing lying here." I told him I'd come back to see him soon. He nodded appreciatively. "Just hearing your voice makes me feel better," he said. "I don't feel so scared." He motioned to John, who was standing beside me, as he had dutifully for the past five years. "You are good men," he said. "I have faith in you. I have faith in what you tell me."

John and I went to the kitchen to speak to his wife. She was sitting silently at the dining table. In the white porcelain sink was a mess of dirty dishes. "He is going to need more Lasix," a diuretic, I told her. She nodded silently, appearing exhausted. I looked in the fridge. It was nearly empty. On the counter there were canned soups, all loaded with sodium, precisely what he should not have been consuming. I told her that I was going to continue the dobutamine, but I didn't want to increase the infusion rate. He was dying, and we all knew it, including him. A visiting nurse was supposed to come by later that day. I left instructions for her to draw blood and fax me the results. Then we bade Elsa goodbye.

We never did make it back to see Mr. Gesselman. For the next couple of weeks we were too busy in the hospital, and he died not long afterward. That house call was our first since I'd started working at LIJ. In 1930, 40 percent of all doctor-patient visits were house calls. Today the proportion has dwindled to less than 1 percent. The major reason, not surprisingly, is money. Traveling to patients' homes is inefficient and almost never profitable. But it felt good to finally do something that didn't have a price tag on it.

After all the wasted time of the past two years, I was eager to focus once again on my heart failure job. I still wanted to create a comprehensive disease management program, implementing best practices into treatment algorithms in the emergency room, on the wards, and in transitional and postdischarge care. Applying such algorithms, I believed, would offer the best chance to reduce hospital costs, readmissions, and mortality. I'd just written a ten-page document summarizing evidence-based practices for heart failure diagnosis and management, which we disseminated to residents and attending physicians. Once I got started, I moved quickly: I audited charts of patients with rapid readmission, hired a case manager to help streamline the transition to outpatient care, began attending multidisciplinary rounds, created a special unit to cluster patients with heart failure diagnoses, partnered with the palliative care service to increase the use of hospice care for my end-stage patients, and took the initial steps to begin an outpatient infusion clinic so that patients who required intravenous medications would not necessarily have to be hospitalized. The lessons I'd learned over five years were with me, and now, finally, I had the time and energy to implement them in practice.

———

Homeostasis is the ability of a biological system to maintain a condition of equilibrium or stability in the face of external stresses. It is closely related to resilience, the power to return to the original form after being bent, compressed, or stretched. In many ways medicine is the study of human resilience—biological, physiological, and emotional—and not just in patients. Perhaps more than any other profession, medicine demands adaptability of its providers.

We start to get bent early on in medicine. In medical school there's the fear factor: Do I know enough to move on to the next stage? The stresses don't end there. In internship and residency there are other pressures, more physical—sleep deprivation, exhaustion—but also existential. And of course, even in full-fledged practice, one is constantly being stretched and bent by factors beyond one's control. There are always new challenges to be faced, no matter which stage you are in on your journey as a doctor, demanding patience and resilience.

How to prevent the burnout that is so widespread in the profession? There are many measures of success in medicine: income, of course, but also creating attachments with patients, making a difference in their lives, providing good care while responsibly managing limited resources. It is whether you find that meaning in your work that determines whether you feel successful or not. The challenge in dealing with physician burnout on a practical level is to create new incentive schemes to foster that meaning: publicizing clinical excellence, for example (of course, we need to better define exactly what that is), or rewarding for patient satisfaction. It won't be easy, but the predominant financial scheme today has created a lot of misery.

In the end, it's a problem of resilience. American doctors need an internal compass to cope with the changing landscape of our profession. For most doctors this compass begins and ends with their patients. In surveys, most physicians—even the dissatisfied ones—say the best part of their jobs is taking care of people. I believe this is the key to coping with the stresses of contemporary medicine: identifying what is important to you, what you believe in, and what you will fight for. For me, I've learned, it's the human moments, such as the house call with Hyman Gesselman. The human moments are what others—the lawyers, the bankers—envy about our profession, and no company, no agency, no entity can take those away.

———

We moved to Long Island on Christmas Eve, a few days before an ice storm. The sunlight that day was blinding, fluorescing off the white world. The moving men showed up early and rapidly disassembled, bundled, packed, and loaded eleven years' worth of our stuff. Standing on the wet sidewalk, I watched the silver Harley from apartment 4E roar out of the garage for the last time. By the time we got on the Long Island Expressway, it was already early afternoon. Dirty spray from the speeding haul truck spattered on my salt-stained windshield. Inside the car, everyone was unusually quiet. I stole furtive glances at Sonia and the children; they were exhausted. I could hardly believe we were finally making our move. It had been a huge decision to uproot my family. I still had no idea if it had been the right one. At our street, tree branches reached out in embrace over the roadway. A sign at the corner said DEAD END.

The house was a white-shingled colonial built in 1955 on a potato farm. In the front yard black locust trees were dusted with white powder, like Christmas cookies. I stepped out of the car. Fresh snow crunched under my feet as we started to unload. On the front porch, icy spears dripped. Inside, the house was empty. We started to sort through our belongings as the kids gingerly explored their new surroundings. I could hear the pitter-patter of Pia's little feet on the bare hardwood floors. As dusk settled, the house got cold and drafty. I convinced the movers to stay for a while; so much work remained to be done. They didn't leave till 10:00 p.m., extorting a huge tip.

I took two weeks off from work to help us get settled. It was a strange and confusing time. We all felt a sense of dislocation, but at times mine seemed overwhelming. (Change always precipitates a measure of fear, whether in the personal or professional realm.) Whenever the kids would cry, I'd feel guilty, as if it were my fault for bringing them there. I imagined Pia missing her stroller ride around our old neighborhood, waving to all the sidewalk fruit vendors. Mohan would call me whenever I went out to run errands after dark, crying, "Dadda, where are you? When are you coming?" Simple tasks like troubleshooting the oven controls or prying open the frozen cover of the trash receptacle left me in a state of panicky frustration. Rajiv, who lived about ten miles away, had his usual no-nonsense take on my gloominess. "How can you compare this house to that apartment in Manhattan?" he demanded. "There is no comparison."

At night the silence was unsettling. I'd sometimes sneak out and gaze up at an owl in the backyard. It was a haunting apparition at the top of a tree, a hooting hole in the fabric of the blue-gray sky. Raccoons scurried off into the bushes, their beady eyes glinting at me through the leafless brush. For months, Mohan would wake up in the middle of the night and call for me. I'd get into bed with him, palming his cranium, pressing it softly. I craved the warmth of his body on those chilly nights, his knee settling comfortably into the small of my back, his sweaty palm tightly clasping my elbow. I slept in his bed as much for me as for him.

One night, while I was lying in his bed, staring up at the fluorescent stars on the ceiling, he asked me, "What if somebody tries to rob a bank in the middle of the night?"

I thought for a moment. "An alarm would go off and the police would come," I said.

"No, they wouldn't. You're just saying that. They couldn't hear it."

Sensing he needed reassurance, I said, "If the alarm goes off, the police get a phone call."

"What if they're sleeping?"

"There's always somebody awake."

"Always?"

"Always."

He sighed, obviously relieved. "Oh, that's good," he said.

Gradually, as the weeks wore on, the pieces of our new lives started to fall into place. We built our first snowman, a grotesque, haphazard sculpture at the base of the driveway. We joined the aquatics program at the Jewish Community Center in Roslyn and started going for family swims on Saturday afternoons. I even restarted my evening runs, sprinting through air crisp and heavy with the fragrance of burning wood. Before long we were shopping for bathroom fixtures at Target on Saturday night. The white fluorescent lights and the immigrant families pushing metal carts transported me back to that time in my life when my parents would pile us all into their beat-up old Buick and take us to Kroger's or Food Town. Buzzed on the scent of fresh-roasted chicken, Rajiv and I would race up and down the aisles with the grocery cart, grabbing boxes of frozen pizzas or TV dinners, tormenting my mother. I missed my parents. Despite all the obstacles they'd faced, they'd succeeded in creating stable and secure lives for their three children. There was a measure of comfort in knowing that I had come full circle, returning to what were more or less my roots.

We were reluctant travelers. We moved to the suburbs because we could no longer afford a certain life in the city. But against all my expectations, it has provided peace of mind, respite from the stresses of urban living, which quelled much of the anxiety I'd been living with. I quickly learned to savor the predictability, the fewer choices, the circumscribed nature of the experience. Just as cells integrate into the matrix in which they land, obeying signals that we can barely fathom, so, too, did we integrate ourselves into our new environment. In fact, I was probably a suburban guy all along. I just hadn't known it.

We enrolled Mohan in a wonderful little school not far from our house. Most mornings I'd drop him off at class, and some afternoons I was even there to greet him at the bus stop. A few weeks after he joined, I ran into one of the school moms at drop-off. "How's it going?" she asked pleasantly.

"Oh, you know, the same," I replied with faux weariness.

She laughed. "Yes, I know. Same thing every day." But I wasn't bothered by the routine, and I suspect neither was she. The routine offered calm and security.

Though we had both grown up in suburbs, Sonia made the move out of the city more gracefully than I did, pulling me along whenever I faltered or lost heart. Perhaps she had been more ready to leave than I'd realized. By springtime she was saying stuff like "It feels like these trees are our friends, even though we cut their limbs off." She made the frequent trips to Home Depot or Britton Hardware to make the house into a home, rushing home to take Mohan to soccer practice, stopping by Whole Foods to pick up groceries or dinner, multitasking constantly.

She also quickly got credentialed at LIJ and started seeing patients. I'd assured her that I would send her referrals, and so would Rajiv and his friends. By then I had learned to accept the referral game. At one time I'd viewed it as a racket to be avoided; now I saw it simply as realpolitik. Insurers can make doctors jump through hoops to get paid. They can tell patients which doctors they can see. They can restrict medications and tests. But they still cannot tell doctors whom or when we can ask for help.

One wine-soaked evening when we were relaxing in front of the fireplace after the kids had gone to bed, Sonia said to me: "Even our bad times have had some good in them. Remember when Mohan was Babydeep?" Her eyes watered, and mine probably did, too. "I've already forgotten. He is so much his own person now."

Later she wrote me this note: "I just wanted to tell you how much I love and adore you. You are EVERYTHING to me: my light, my hope, my best friend in this funny journey. I think what I've always loved about you is how you always have long pieces of black curly hair falling over your prominent and shiny forehead. Little Mohan isn't there . . . yet." Relaxing that night amid bookshelves in the armchair in my tiny den, my kids in their animal pajamas asleep in their beds, I felt a contentment that had been missing for too long.

———

Rajiv invited me to join his tennis group. They hit every Sunday morning at an indoor tennis complex in Huntington, a community of steeple churches and conservancies about ten miles from where I lived. The first time I played with them was a few weeks after we moved. I left the house at 7:00 a.m. and nearly slipped on the front steps. The frigid air burned my bare legs. The wipers on my car were stuck, so I turned on the defroster and waited for the ice to melt. (Be patient, you cannot rush it. Things don't happen immediately.) Gradually the car warmed up, and the frozen sheet on the windshield shattered into countless pieces.

Joggers in polychromatic Gore-Tex were out on the slushy road. I sped up Northern Boulevard, past the docks in Cold Spring Harbor, past the golf courses and plant nurseries and estates sequestered by iron gates and pointy yew hedges. Walking trails branched out from the roadway, ducking into the snow-shrouded woods. When I arrived at the court, Matt, a stent salesman at Medtronic and a former college player, was feeding balls to Rajiv and three of his doctor friends: Chaudhry, Gupta, and Goldner. "Nice shot, Confucius," Rajiv called out to Gupta, a cardiologist in private practice, who was growing a beard. Gupta reached to hit a low backhand volley, which he dumped into the middle of the net. "For a man, you bend over well," Rajiv taunted. Then he hit a passing shot. "There you go, baby. Can't touch this!"

Matt was lobbing balls to Chaudhry. "No overheads," Chaudhry protested. "My back is too stiff." He was an enthusiastic, if stodgy, player, with the slightly awkward strokes of someone who had picked up the game as an adult. He turned his shoulders to protect his back, ironically just the right move to allow him to line up the shot perfectly. "Do that every time and you'll be fine," Matt told him.

Already drenched in sweat, Gupta came over to rest on the bench where I was stretching. Rajiv held up his hand to stop play. "Let up on him, Matt," he said, grinning wickedly. "I'm on interventional call. If he has a heart attack, I'm going to have to leave."

I took Gupta's place on the court. Everyone greeted me pleasantly, though I could tell that Chaudhry was a bit uncomfortable with my being there. "All right, it's the Jauhar brothers," Matt announced as I hopped up and down at the baseline to warm up. "Let's get some good old-fashioned competition going. I know Sandeep is not going to want to lose to your ass."

Soon I was sliding from side to side on the Har-Tru as Matt fed us balls. Though I'd played a lot in high school and occasionally on weekends since moving to New York, my strokes were off, and I was hopelessly out of shape. "Move to the ball!" Matt commanded. "One bounce, one bounce!" After long rallies I'd crouch at the baseline, panting. Matt came over and instructed me on the proper form for my backhand. "Follow through," he said, extending my arms upward. "Never stop in the middle. When you stop halfway, that's the worst thing you can do."

After about fifteen minutes of intense workout, my back started to spasm, and I had to lie down on the side of the court to ease the tightness. Gupta held up my legs, angling them to stretch the muscle, as I tried in vain to dodge the bullets dripping off his chin. "You've got to stretch more," he said, while the others kept playing. He told me he did kung fu to stay fit. Crouching beside me, he told me to throw a punch at him, which he easily slapped away. Then his hands went into a rapid circular motion, and before I could say anything, his right hand had grabbed my throat. "See, that's how a tiger moves," he said proudly. "You should try it sometime."

When the hour was up, the others shuffled off the court. I overheard Rajiv and Chaudhry talking business on the sidelines. "It's forty percent overhead, boss . . . no, we can get you the space. The tech will come in, but you need to establish the accreditation . . ." They walked up to where the rest of us were.

"When I leave here, I always tell myself I'm going to get into shape," Rajiv said.

Goldner added: "Mine is the opposite reaction. I feel like I've gotten my exercise for the month."

We started to gather up our wallets, watches, BlackBerrys, and beepers.

Matt surveyed the accessories. "Take a picture of this, guys," he said. "This is our lives."

Rajiv slung his tennis bag over his shoulder. Pointing at Matt, he said to me, "He's having a midlife crisis, too. What do you always say, Matt?"

"The older I get, the better I used to be." Everyone laughed.

Rajiv and I walked out together to our cars. I told him that Sonia and I were planning our first dinner party for physicians. He quipped, "If you don't get at least a couple of referrals out of it, it's a waste of time." I asked him how Chaudhry was doing. "The same," Rajiv replied. "He says every day is a headache. He's thinking about taking on another gig, reading studies for some doctor named Hasani."

"Hasani?" I was nonplussed. "I thought Chaudhry hated Hasani."

"Who's going to turn down a chance to make more money?"

"When you're making as much as he is?"

"It doesn't matter how much you make. Most people want to make more."

———

One night in Mohan's room, I banged my knee on his bedpost and cried out in pain. Later he asked me why dads don't cry.

"Sometimes we do," I said.

"When?"

"Like when we're happy. Like the first time you scored a goal in soccer, I got a tear in my eye."

"What about when you get hurt?"

"Not so much."

"Why?"

"I don't know. The tears get dried when you get older."

"Do you try to cry?"

"No, but even if we did, the tears wouldn't come out."

"Because you use up all the tears in your tear ducts?" he said, showing off some knowledge he'd acquired.

"Yeah, I guess so," I replied, chuckling.

"That's good," he said, settling into his pillow.

I put on a Beatles song, as I often did when putting him to bed.

"This song reminds me of going to the park in New York," he said.

"Yeah, when we were lying on the grass. Do you remember?"

"Yes."

"Do you miss the park?"

He thought for a moment. "Not really."

I felt relieved. "This song reminds me of when I was younger," I said.

"When?"

"When I was in college, before you were born."

"Before I was born?"

"Yeah, I wasn't always your dad."

For a moment he didn't say anything. Then he said, "Did you want me to be a boy or a girl?"

I laughed. "I wanted a boy. And I got you. I didn't just get a boy; I got the best boy."

He smiled. I switched off the light. We were lying in the dark. "Dad?"

"Yeah."

"If you're bored, instead of putting me to bed, you can just go do your computer."

"That's okay, Mohan, I like putting you to bed. Remember when I never had time to do that?"

"Now you do it all the time."

"Well, I love spending time with you."

"I love spending time with you, too, Dad."

He turned and put his hand on my shoulder. I stroked his head and told him to go to sleep.

———

The Huntington Historical Society was doing an exhibit about Long Island medicine. It was in an old farmhouse on a quiet street of quaint shops and galleries not far from where I played tennis. The exhibit featured a former chief of obstetrics at Huntington Hospital named Samuel Teich. Born and educated in Huntington, he joined the army in 1940 and landed at Normandy on D-day, for which he was awarded the Bronze Star for bravery. When he came home from the war, he hung up a shingle in Huntington Station and started a private practice. He became the chief surgeon of the Huntington Police Department and eventually the chief obstetrician at Huntington Hospital, which had opened its doors only three decades earlier.

Teich's career spanned an era of great change in medicine. A big shift, thanks to the GI Bill, was the rise of specialists. In 1940, three-quarters of America's physicians were general practitioners, but by 1960 specialists outnumbered generalists, and by 1970 only a quarter of doctors counted themselves general practitioners. (Today the trend away from primary care continues, threatening access to care for millions of Americans.) Physicians' average salary (corrected for inflation) increased dramatically over this period, too, and the average net profit from private practice quadrupled. This increase paralleled an equally dramatic rise in national medical expenses, from $3 billion in 1940 to $75 billion in 1970.

The venue of care also shifted. In 1930, 40 percent of encounters between doctors and patients took place in patients' homes. By 1960 that number had dropped to 10 percent. In 1935 half of all births presided over by doctors were home births. Twenty years later, only 4 percent of all births took place at home. In the early 1930s, only one physician in sixteen worked in a hospital full-time. Today that number is more than 50 percent and rising as hospitals and health systems, eager to acquire more leverage in negotiating contracts with insurers, rapaciously buy up private practices.

Perhaps the biggest change has been in the doctor-patient relationship. The exhibit showed a replica of Teich's examination room, like my grandfather's, with old-fashioned instruments, evoking a bygone era: an exam table with wooden stirrups, a cystoscope, a hemometer for estimating blood counts, an old-style wicker baby scale. There were photographs of Dr. Teich with nurses in white vestments and white hats. On display were Christmas cards with pictures of some of the ten thousand babies Teich had delivered, some spanning three generations. But most striking were the scores of patient testimonials. "We shall always remember you as a friend, and it is a privilege to know you," a patient wrote. "Some Saturday we shall grace your office just to say hello. We have planned that for a long time, but it is not so easy to borrow a car." Another said: "I am enclosing a check in your favor for the amount of one hundred dollars, as an additional payment on account of the services you rendered us and for which your statement has never been received.

I have no idea of the actual amount in dollars and cents, but I am convinced that any further payments that may be required to balance the books would indeed be a very poor substitute for the feeling of gratitude that we bear toward you." And another (in May 1964): "Words are inadequate. My husband and I were heartbroken when we lost the other baby, but now we have a beautiful, bouncing baby boy. You were so kind and thoughtful all through my pregnancy that I felt I just had to say thank you again."

Doctors in Teich's era, practicing on the heels of revolutionary medical advances, commanded unusual respect and influence. However, as Dr. Abigail Zuger argues in a 2004 article in *The New England Journal of Medicine*, this golden era was probably an aberration. Several nineteenth-century American doctors wrote in their memoirs of their fathers' "contempt" and "disgust" on learning that they had decided to enter medicine. One doctor, writing in a medical journal in 1869, called medicine "the most despised of all the professions" for educated men. At the beginning of the twentieth century, medical education was not standardized. Quacks routinely cut into doctors' business. In 1913 the American Medical Association estimated that no more than 10 percent of physicians were able to earn a comfortable living. "A doctor's life is made up of moments of terrible nervous tension," wrote a physician in the early twentieth century. "There are times when the powers to continue such a life are entirely exhausted and you are seized with such depression that only one thought remains—to turn your back on all and flee."

Gauging our professional lives by the short-lived golden era of medicine is a bit like judging a marriage by a honeymoon. Expectations are impossibly high, a recipe for dissatisfaction. Fulfillment in medicine, as with any endeavor, is about managing hopes. Probably the group best equipped to deal with the changes racking the profession today is medical students because they are not so weighed down by their expectations. It is the doctors ensconced in professional midlife who are having the hardest time. Of course, there are many factions to blame for the state of American medicine—insurers, malpractice lawyers, the federal government—but doctors must take a hard look at themselves, too. Managed care alone didn't create medicine's midlife crisis. Indeed, this crisis was also spurred by the abandonment of professional ideals in the pursuit of profit that made managed care necessary in the first place.

———

Today I am living my life in archetypal roles: often doting father, occasionally reserved husband, at times discouraged doctor. There are recurring patterns in our lives, in the characters that we play. In thermodynamics the triple point of a substance is that temperature and pressure where three phases (gas, solid, and liquid) coexist. This feels like the point I am at in my midlife: husband, doctor, father—all in uneasy equilibrium. I am learning to be more modest in my expectations and more humble in my ignorance. Like my father, I have begun to appreciate that the old wisdom has a lot to offer.

Of course, I wish I'd more consistently lived up to my youthful ideals. I've made the same compromises that Rajiv, Chaudhry, and others have made and continue to make. But tolerance develops for life's circumstances, especially if they develop slowly. In congestive heart failure, if cardiac pressure increases gradually, the left atrium enlarges and becomes more compliant, thus able to accommodate the increased volume of blood. It is only when the pressure increases rapidly that the patient crashes and burns.

I see a glimmer that these middle years will make me stronger, that eventually I'll master my most difficult experiences and look back on them like a vivid dream. Yet it still feels at times as if I am running in place, like one of Chaudhry's patients trying to keep up with the treadmill. So I will muddle through this period, trying to find peace with the changes that are occurring. I have already mostly forgotten the pain of my internship. All I have now is the memory of that time, and it doesn't seem so awful. Perhaps all this will blow over, too, and I will be able to revise in my mind how I felt about it.

What kind of doctor do you want to be? This is a question that all physicians have to answer at various points in their careers. And they have to do it with the knowledge that people often place outsize expectations on our profession. People often think of doctors as either consumedly avaricious or impossibly altruistic. There is a disconnect between how the lay world views medicine and how doctors experience it from the inside.

One weekend when I was on call in the ICU as a second-year resident, I was on rounds with Abe Sanders, the attending. Dr. Sanders was a portly, avuncular man with a mischievous grin. Despite the miseries of the ICU, he always maintained a relentlessly upbeat manner.

It was a brilliantly sunny day, perfect weather for sailing. Midway through long, protracted rounds, Sanders called us over to a window. He pointed down at a sailboat on the river. A man was standing on the deck, looking up at the hospital. He looked as if he were about Sanders's age, though fit and tan. He was holding a drink, and a party with attractive people was being held on board. "See that guy?" Sanders said. "Do you know what he's thinking?"

We were standing in a patient's room. The alarms were going off. No one ventured a guess.

Sanders said: "He's thinking, 'I should have been a doctor!'"

Of course, I now have a much more nuanced view of medicine than the man on the boat. Having been in medicine for the better part of my professional life, I have seen that there are all types: knights, knaves, and pawns. In fact, most doctors—myself included—are an amalgam of all three. Neither we nor the profession in which we practice is perfect.

Still, I believe most doctors continue to want to be knights. Most of us went into medicine to help people, not to follow corporate directives or to maximize income. We want to practice medicine the right way, but too many forces today are propelling us away from the bench or the bedside. No one ever goes into medicine to do unnecessary testing. However, this sort of behavior is rampant. The American system too often seems to promote knavery over knighthood.

But medicine holds the key to its own redemption. A few years ago there was an intern, Jeremy, at my hospital who started his residency when he was forty-six years old. He had gone to medical school in his twenties, but midway through his fourth year he developed lymphoma. He'd been forced to forgo residency. He'd gone into medical education instead, and eventually worked his way to becoming a top-level administrator, the chief operating officer of a large hospital system in Philadelphia, commanding a high six-figure salary and a staff of six assistants. One day I asked him, "What the hell were you thinking when you decided to quit that and become an intern?"

This is what he said to me. "I hit the big forty-five and asked myself, What is this? What am I doing? I had always just wanted to practice medicine." So he started going on rounds at 6:00 a.m. daily with an

ICU team at one of the hospitals he was overseeing. "I loved being there," he said. "I just wanted to be taking care of people."

In the middle of his second year at LIJ, he suffered another health setback—a new primary bladder cancer for which he had to undergo chemotherapy—and yet he persevered and applied for a fellowship in critical care medicine, eventually going to the Mayo Clinic in Rochester, Minnesota. "I've had a great time," he told me when he graduated. He didn't seem fazed by his health condition or by the fact that he was going to be fifty-one years old when he finally finished his medical training.

I believe most people who are drawn to medicine desire a career of tangible purpose, like Jeremy. What redeems the effort? It's the tender moments helping people in need. In the end, medicine is about taking care of people in their most vulnerable state and making yourself a bit of the same in the process. When I get dispirited, I often think of my eighty-eight-year-old patient Lily Dunhill standing at the doorway to my office. "I'm sorry to bother you, Doctor, but can I share with you a thought? It's sort of my philosophy on life." I looked up from my keyboard, where I was tapping out my report on her. "When you get to be my age, you don't want to take life too seriously. You know the old saying: If you laugh, the whole world will laugh with you. Well, I say, When you cry, your mascara runs." She smiled warmly. "Thank you for being a good and kind doctor. What you're doing is so, so important."

Epilogue

A buzzing on my waist. I pull off my beeper. The teal display lights up in the dark. I reach for the phone. There is perspiration on the back of my neck.

"Dr. Chaudhry's service," a woman says.

"This is Dr. Jauhar," I whisper.

"The ER just paged again, Doctor. About Martha Reed."

"How is it they called again? I just talked to them."

"I'm sorry, Doctor. Can I connect you?"

I stare into the dark. Sonia is fast asleep. A soporific buzz rises from the vent.

"Doctor?"

"Yes, go ahead."

I pull myself up and step out of the bedroom. It is 3:00 a.m. The floorboards creak noisily, as if complaining, too, of being woken. I go downstairs. Through a living room window the moon is shining brightly. Shadows of trees slice across the lawn. The white hydrangeas are glowing like tiny orbs of light.

"LIJ ER," a voice announces.

"Yes, it's Dr. Jauhar, doc-of-the-day."

"Hold on, Dr. Jauhar." In the darkness of the living room, I stare at the mantelpiece. The nocturnal feeling that the ER is being unfair to me is beginning to take hold. After a minute—maybe more, I don't know—the receptionist finally comes back on the phone. "Dr. Jauhar, I went round and round, but nobody's owning up to it. Maybe it's a page from earlier."

"No, the answering service just called me. Can you check again? I don't know why you guys can't coordinate your calls. I've gotten six phone calls—"

"I'm sorry, Dr. Jauhar. Hold on."

Another minute passes. The room is pretty, though unfinished. Swatches of fabric lie on the rug. Finally a voice says, "Dr. Jauhar, it's Sabrina, telemetry PA. The family wants to know if they can take Martha Reed home. They say she has a history of infectious colitis, and they're concerned she's going to get it again."

"Then why did they bring her to the hospital?"

"I really don't know, Dr. Jauhar. I wish I could tell you . . . Dr. Jauhar?"

I must have dozed off. "Yes, well, I can't let her leave. I'll talk to them in the morning."

"Okay, Dr. Jauhar. I'll tell them. While I have you on the phone, can I tell you about this other patient, Rita Roberts? She is forty years old. She's been having mild chest pain for four months, no relation with exertion, comes and goes. No cardiac risk factors, but her outside attending wants her to have an angiogram. So I'm going to call the fellow for a consult."

I try to focus, but my mind is a blur. Perhaps I should intervene, question the rationale of sending a healthy woman with atypical chest pain for cardiac catheterization, protest the risks that we were going to force this young woman to endure. Perhaps I should call her doctor and demand to know why after four months of symptoms he thinks it is warranted to spend thousands of dollars admitting her to the hospital to do an unnecessary procedure—on my watch. But I say nothing. I will deal with it in the morning.

Notes

2. ODD CONCEPTIONS

48 *encouraging a kind of shiftwork mentality* I have worked in teaching hospitals in
New York State for fifteen years, first as a resident and now as an attending physician, mentoring residents and fellows. Over this period I have discerned a gradual
decline in the intellectual climate of these institutions. It has been dispiriting to
watch. Of all the places one might expect doctors to be curious about medicine,
teaching hospitals should be first.

I once met a pulmonologist, a soft-spoken woman who told me that she used
to work on the staff of a teaching hospital in New York City but had gone into
private practice a few years before. I asked her why. "I loved to teach," she replied
sadly, "but the residents and fellows just didn't seem to want to learn. They had
other things on their minds.

"I met an intern the other day," she went on. "He was asking me questions
about a case we were managing together. I told him that it was wonderful to see
a young doctor so curious about medicine. He said: 'Thank you for saying so.
Now can you tell my chiefs because they are always telling me that I am too
inefficient?'"

In his 1999 book *Time to Heal: American Medical Education from the Turn of
the Century to the Era of Managed Care*, Kenneth Ludmerer, a Washington University physician and historian, bemoans the deteriorating intellectual environment in teaching hospitals.

He writes: "Most pernicious of all from the standpoint of education, house
officers"—interns and residents—"to a considerable extent were reduced to workup machines and disposition-arrangers: admitting patients and planning their
discharge, one after another, with much less time than before to examine them,
confer with attending physicians, teach medical students, attend conferences,
read the literature and reflect and wonder."

5. DO THE RIGHT THING

91 *and many more lives were at stake* A decade ago the Office of the City Comptroller of New York City issued a troubling report that found that volunteer ambulances were apparently biased toward transporting patients to the hospitals that hired them, even if it meant delaying taking patients to the ER or passing other hospitals along the way. At the time, Alan Hevesi, the comptroller, said that volunteer ambulances sometimes "put the financial interest of their hospitals ahead of the health of patients."

102 *the models did not account for simple bad luck* Any doctor dreads bad luck, but for cardiac surgeons, who generally perform no more than a couple of hundred operations a year, it can be ruinous. A few unexpected outcomes can wreak havoc on a surgeon's statistics. This point was illustrated in an elegant 1977 article in *Scientific American*, in which the mathematicians Bradley Efron and Carl Morris studied the batting averages of eighteen Major League baseball players after their first forty-five at bats during the 1970 baseball season. Using statistical arguments, they showed that the batting average of any player converges to the mean batting average of all players if he takes a sufficient number of swings. That is, the true ability of a batter is not what you observe after a small number of at bats because a handful of strikeouts can ruin a batter's average. The smaller the number of at bats, the greater the potential deviation from that player's "true" average. This "regression to the mean" can just as well be applied to cardiac surgeons, for whom a few deaths can be statistically ruinous. More important, it calls into question the validity of statistically guided surgical quality-improvement programs.

8. PACT

139 *that would be a bad thing* A recent study of 250 high-billing physicians found that those doctors did not perform 66 percent of their billed procedures. More troubling, 21 percent of procedures were performed by "unqualified" staff.

14. DECEPTION

203 *made fainting seem benign, almost glamorous* The common faint—or vasovagal syncope—accounts for roughly three-quarters of the cases of syncope that come through the emergency room. A grab-bag diagnosis, it is probably not a single disease as much as a poorly understood syndrome of standing. The classic physical signs are slow pulse and low blood pressure. A cardiologist once told me how he had diagnosed vasovagal syncope on a plane flight. A passenger in the aisle had started to pass out, and as he was falling, the cardiologist's fingers somehow had landed on his neck pulse, which was beating slowly. Given the circumstances, it was all he'd needed to make the diagnosis. Rarely fatal, vasovagal syncope can be debilitating to those predisposed. Treatment suggestions reflect the

wide spectrum of the disorder, ranging from beta-blocking drugs and salt tablets to pacemakers and Paxil.

16. FOLLOW THE MONEY

228 *such "gainsharing" will align physicians' incentives with cost-cutting goals* In 2009, CMS announced a gainsharing demonstration project at twelve New Jersey hospitals that offers doctors financial rewards for helping the hospitals improve efficiency and lower costs by reducing length of stay, improving discharge planning, and so on. There are safeguards in the program to ensure that quality of care does not suffer. This project, one of many piloted under health care reform legislation, is a step in the right direction. Unless doctors view cost-cutting goals as their own, policy makers don't stand a chance of achieving them.

Acknowledgments

There are many people I wish to thank for their help and support during the writing of this book.

First and foremost, I am deeply indebted to the patients I've had the privilege of caring for and learning from during my years as an attending physician. My relationships with you have enriched my life in more ways than I can enumerate.

My agent, Todd Shuster, has been a friend and advocate for fifteen years. I am grateful for his perseverance and faith.

Most authors would be lucky to have one great editor. I had three. Paul Elie, a brilliant writer himself, had a clear vision for this book and urged me to write it. His successor, Courtney Hodell, astutely shepherded the manuscript through a first draft. And finally, the preternaturally smart Alex Star helped me mold the book into its current form. Alex's fine editorial touches are present on nearly every page. I feel so incredibly fortunate to have had the opportunity to work with him.

I am also thankful for the assistance of several other colleagues at Farrar, Straus, and Giroux: Laird Gallagher, who attended to so many important details during the course of this enterprise; Taylor Sperry, who read through the first draft and made numerous helpful suggestions; Susan Goldfarb, my wonderful production editor; and Katie Kurtzman, my publicist.

And of course I am indebted to Jonathan Galassi for giving me the chance to write the book in the first place.

I have had the enormous privilege of writing for *The New York Times* for almost two decades. I am grateful to the many editors who have helped shape me into a writer, but I owe a special thanks to David Corcoran, who edited some of the journalism that made its way into the book.

Medicine and writing are distinct but complementary spheres in my professional life. I am extraordinarily lucky to have such a tremendous group of colleagues at Long Island Jewish Medical Center, where I work. John Meister has been a loyal comrade for nearly a decade. Janine Sandy, my assistant, keeps my workday running smoothly. I owe a special thanks to Stacey Rosen, my chief during the years I was writing this book, as well as to my current bosses, Stanley Katz and Barry Kaplan, for their ongoing support. I am also grateful for the extraordinarily industrious cardiology fellows I work with. You make my job easy.

I also wish to acknowledge several in the leadership of the North Shore–LIJ Health System who have been encouraging of my work, including Michael Dowling, David Battinelli, and Lawrence Smith, Dean of the Hofstra North Shore–LIJ School of Medicine, who offered me one of my most rewarding roles: teaching cardiology to first-year medical students.

Several other colleagues have earned my heartfelt appreciation, including David Slotwiner, Maya Frankfurt, Jacob Moore, and Danielle Ofri, who all critiqued early drafts of the manuscript, and Sheena Gupta, who assisted me with the research.

Of course, the narrative has relied on my memory of events that in some cases occurred a decade ago. If my memory has failed me, the fault is mine and mine alone.

I save my deepest gratitude for my family: my parents, Prem and Raj, and my sister, Suneeta. My brother, Rajiv, stands out for special recognition. He read through many drafts of the manuscript and generally was an unflagging reservoir of support throughout the entire enterprise. No words can repay my debt to him. I am also obliged to my father-in-law, Madho Sharma, for his generosity and backing.

Parenthood is the best part of my existence. I want to recognize the twin lights of my life: my son, Mohan, my best friend and right-hand man, and my darling little girl, Pia, who was just a baby as this project was taking off and provided the hugs and kisses that helped to pull me away from it. I hope one day they will read this book and be as proud of me as I am of them.

Finally, I am so grateful to my wife, Sonia, for being my life partner and gracing me with all the things that add up to a special life. This book would not exist without her, and so it is only fitting that I end it with her.